Drug and Alcohol Abuse

The Authoritative Guide for Parents, Teachers, and Counselors

H. Thomas Milhorn, Jr., M.D., Ph.D.

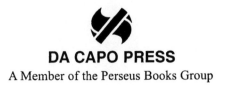

DA CAPO PRESS

A Member of the Perseus Books Group

Jacket design by Suzanne Van Duyne

Cataloging in Publication data is available from the Library of Congress.

First Da Capo Press paperback edition 2003
First published in the United States by Perseus Books (U.S.)
This edition published by arrangement with the author.
ISBN 0–306–81324–6

Published by Da Capo Press
A Member of the Perseus Books Group
http://www.dacapopress.com

Da Capo Press books are available at special discounts for bulk purchases in the U.S. by corporations, institutions, and other organizations. For more information, please contact the Special Markets Department at the Perseus Books Group, 11 Cambridge Center, Cambridge, MA 02142, or call (800) 255-1514 or (617) 252-5298, or e-mail j.mccrary@perseusbooks.com.

3   4   5   6   7   8   9   10—06   05   04   03

Preface

Abuse of alcohol and other drugs has reached epidemic proportions in the United States. The "war on drugs" quite clearly has been less than effective. The time has come for parents, teachers, and counselors to take matters into their own hands. Prevention remains the only true hope for solving our nation's drug problem. Parents, teachers, and counselors are in the best positions to affect children's knowledge and attitudes about the abuse of alcohol and other drugs. Waiting for others, such as school administrations, communities, or governments, to do the job will only increase the risk that children become drug addicted.

Before teaching children about drugs, you must first educate yourself. Children have little difficulty perceiving who is a credible speaker and who is not. In this book you will find important information on the classification of drugs of abuse, how drugs of abuse differ from other drugs, alcoholism as a disease, why adolescents abuse drugs, how to prevent drug abuse, how to tell if your child is abusing drugs, what you can do if your child is abusing drugs, what goes on in treatment, special issues of young women, what help is available for the rest of the family, what to expect when your child comes home from treatment, what to do if he or she uses drugs again, whether drug abuse causes mental problems, how drug abuse and AIDS are related, and whether you have issues of your own on which you need to work. In addition, the pharmacology of drugs of abuse, as well as their histories, actions, abstinence syndromes, and health consequences are discussed.

One appendix contains information on where to get help or information, a second contains recommended reading for children, a third contains sources of videos for parents and teachers, and a glossary presents common terminology and definitions. In addition, recommended reading for teachers, parents, and counselors is indicated in the references.

I thank Lyndell Gardner for typing the manuscript; my wife, Kay, for encouraging me to write it; and my son, Toby, for being drug free.

H. Thomas Milhorn, Jr.

Contents

I. Background

Appendixes

I

Background

1

Introduction

THE PROBLEM

The average ages of first alcohol use and first illicit drug use in the United States are 12 and 13 years, respectively. Well over one-half of American high school seniors have tried an illicit drug, and over one-third have used an illicit drug other than marijuana; nearly one in six seniors has tried cocaine. High school girls come close to the level of boys in their use of alcohol, marijuana, and cocaine. Close to one-half of 4th through 6th graders report pressure from other students to try alcohol, and over one-fourth of these children say there is pressure to try cocaine.

Accidents is the leading cause of death among adolescents. Of the 25,000 accidental deaths among them annually, 40 percent are alcohol related. Homicide is the second leading cause of adolescent deaths. Of the 5500 adolescent homicide victims each year, 30 percent are intoxicated at the time of death. The suicide rate among drug-using adolescents is particularly high. Overall, drug abuse is one of the leading, if not the leading, cause of adolescent deaths. Less dramatic, but more insidious, are the developmental, emotional, and social costs of adolescent drug abuse.

Parents, teachers, and counselors have special opportunities to positively affect children's knowledge and attitudes about the abuse of alcohol and other drugs.

WHAT EVERY PARENT, TEACHER, AND COUNSELOR SHOULD KNOW

Every parent, teacher, and counselor should know the answers to these 15 questions about drug abuse:

1. What are drugs of abuse?
2. How do drugs of abuse differ from other drugs?
3. Is alcoholism truly a disease?
4. Why do adolescents abuse drugs?
5. Can drug abuse be prevented?
6. How can I tell if my child is abusing drugs?
7. What can I do if my child is abusing drugs?
8. What does treatment entail?
9. Do young women have special issues?
10. What help can be provided for the rest of the family?
11. What happens when my child comes home from treatment?
12. What can I do if he or she uses drugs again?
13. Does drug abuse cause mental problems?
14. How are drug abuse and AIDS related?
15. Do I have problems of my own which I need to work on?

Throughout this book you will learn the crucial answers to these questions and more.*

BASIC DEFINITIONS

A *psychoactive substance* is defined as a chemical that exerts a mood altering effect on the brain and which is capable of producing addiction. The terms *psychoactive substance* and *drug*, or *drug of abuse*, are used interchangeably. The term *drug* includes alcohol. The terms *addiction* and *dependence* are also used interchangeably.

---

*For the sake of simplicity, I will use "he" throughout the text to refer to children.

Dependence is the medical term for what is commonly called addiction. Chemical dependence is a term used to connote addiction to alcohol and/or other drugs.

A drug which, on stopping its use, causes withdrawal symptoms is said to produce *physical dependence*. A drug which, on stopping its use, does not cause withdrawal symptoms is said to produce *psychological dependence*. Withdrawal symptoms are also known as *abstinence syndrome*.

With prolonged use, more and more of the drug becomes needed to get the same effect, a phenomenon known as *tolerance*. The development of tolerance to drugs within the same group as an abused drug, *cross-tolerance*, can occur without actual use of the other drugs. Heroin addicts, for example, develop tolerance to morphine, although they may never have used it.

Cross-addiction means that a person who has been addicted to one drug can never use any drug without serious risk of becoming addicted to that drug. An alcoholic, for example, having given up alcohol, cannot switch to cocaine without serious risk of becoming addicted to it.

An *addict* is defined as a person who is presently, or has been in the past, addicted to one or more drugs. It is customary to divide addicts into those whose addiction involves alcohol (*alcoholic*) and those whose addiction involves other drugs (*drug addict*). In reality, most addicts use both alcohol and other drugs. An addict living a life of sobriety is said to be in *recovery*.

PROGRESSION TO ADDICTION

All adolescents who use drugs do not become addicted; some try them and do not like them. Some use them nonaddictively for years and eventually stop. Others, however, become hopelessly addicted. The progression from drug use to drug addiction develops continuously over a period of time, usually months to years. It is convenient, however, to categorize this process into three separate but somewhat arbitrary stages—use, abuse, and addiction.

Use

Drug use commonly begins in adolescence, usually with nicotine from cigarettes, and often progresses from nicotine to the use of alcohol and illicit drugs.

Initially, drug use is limited to weekends. Later, however, use may begin to take place during the week, but only in the evenings. Adolescents learn that the drug will provide the feeling they desire and that it will provide it every time. They learn to control the degree of this feeling by regulating the amount of drug they use. At this point they can either take the drug or leave it. Since drug use usually takes place with friends, this stage is sometimes referred to as *social use*.

Abuse

In this stage, the frequency of drug use increases. Adolescents begin to maintain their own supplies, and may begin to use drugs when alone rather than with friends. Drug use, however, continues to take place mainly in the evenings and on weekends. Users can still control the time, the amount, and the circumstances of their drug use. They rarely show up at school or at home intoxicated. Adolescents in this stage develop some degree of tolerance, so they have to increase the quantity of drug they use to get the same effect. They may have occasionally minor conflicts with parents, school officials, and the police.

Addiction

In this stage, adolescents use drugs every day, or nearly so. They begin to use them during the weekdays as well as in the evenings and on weekends. Tolerance develops to the point where large quantities of drugs are required to get "high." *Blackouts* (not remembering what one did when under the influence of a drug) begin to occur and become more frequent. Users now prefer to use drugs by themselves rather than with friends, and drugs become the main focus of their lives, which revolve around getting, keeping, and using drugs. Almost all activities involve drugs and drug-using friends. They no longer have nonusing friends. When confronted by family members or friends, they deny that their drug use is a problem. Family relationships, school performance, and health progressively deteriorate. Adolescents in this stage may be arrested for driving under the influence, possessing controlled substances, drunk and disorderly conduct, or even dealing drugs.

Withdrawal symptoms occur with many drugs if adolescents stop using them in this stage, and users experience severe craving for the drug. They now have to use drugs just to feel normal. *Loss of control* occurs; that is, the addicted adolescent is not always able to stop using the drug once he begins. The compulsion to use the drug is overwhelming. Drug use continues despite adverse consequences. Adolescents deny to themselves and to others that the adverse consequences are the result of their drug use.

Many authorities, including the American Society of Addiction Medicine, do not recognize abuse as a separate stage. They consider what we have called abuse to be early addiction. I shall consider it as early addiction in the remainder of this book.

Crossing the Wall

Progression from use to addiction is often referred to as *crossing the wall* (Fig. 1). In the use stage, the adolescent can cut back or stop using the drug as situations dictate. Once he or she becomes addicted to the drug, however, trying to quit using it is no longer a matter of choice. Attempts to quit using the drug in this stage are said to resemble beating your head against a brick wall. It is very hard to do without outside help. The progression from use to addiction—dependence—occurs much more rapidly in adolescents than in adults, a phenomenon known as *telescoping*.

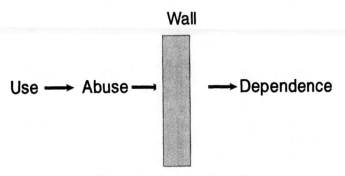

Figure 1.1. Crossing the wall.

The reason for this is uncertain but may relate to the fact that the adolescent brain is in a developmental stage.

CAUSE OF DRUG ADDICTION

The reason why some adolescents who use drugs become addicted to them and others do not is unclear. Theories abound. Most of these theories can be categorized into a *biological model*, a *psychological model*, a *social model*, and a *disease model*.

Biological Model

The biological model argues that people who become addicted to drugs are in some way biologically different from people who do not become addicted to them. This factor, whatever it is, is thought to make some individuals more susceptible to becoming addicted than others. Evidence from studies of twins and adopted children of alcoholic fathers strongly suggests that genetic predisposition is a contributing factor, at least in alcoholics.

Studies of alcoholism in twins have shown that if one identical twin (same genetic makeup) is alcoholic, the other twin has about a 50 percent chance of also being alcoholic. On the other hand, if a nonidentical twin (not the same genetic makeup) is alcoholic, the other twin has only about a 25 percent chance of being alcoholic. Thus, having an identical genetic makeup as an alcoholic puts one at greater risk of becoming alcoholic than having a different genetic makeup. Furthermore, male adopted children who have alcoholic natural fathers are almost four times as likely to become alcoholic as male adopted children who do not have alcoholic fathers. Thus, alcoholism cannot be explained on an environmental basis alone. On the other hand, a significant number of people who do not have an alcoholic parent (no genetic disposition) also develop alcoholism, indicating that although genetic makeup may make it easier to become alcoholic, it is not a required condition. Studies are in progress to determine if genetic dispositions also occur for other drugs of abuse.

Psychological Model

The psychological model argues that certain personality types, personality traits, or other abnormal psychological states predispose individuals to becoming addicted. Underlying emotional states are thought to be relieved by drug use. Drug use is viewed, therefore, as a form of self-medication. It is considered to be only symptomatic of an underlying psychological disorder. According to this model, drug use would be expected to stop once its cause had been effectively treated; however, studies looking at personality characteristics have shown little or no difference between individuals who later become addicted to drugs and those who do not. Personality characteristics of individuals in recovery also do not vary significantly from those who have never been addicted to drugs. In short, there is no such thing as an addictive personality, except during the time individuals are actively using drugs.

Social Model

The social model argues that substance abuse is learned from environmental influences and experiences, much in the same way that language and social customs are learned. Drug abuse is considered to be controlled by external, environmental stimuli, such as underemployment, poverty, family discord, and job or school stress. The social model has difficulty explaining drug addiction in middle class and upper class individuals. While children growing up in drug-using families and those who undergo intensive peer pressure to use drugs are more likely to initiate drug use, why some go on to become addicted and others do not is not explained by this model.

Disease Model

Because drug addiction is a pathological state with characteristic signs and symptoms and a predictable course and outcome if untreated, most authorities consider it to be a disease state. This model considers drug addiction to involve an interplay among all three factors—psychological, social, and biological. Thus, it is considered to be a *biopsychosocial disease*. It is characterized by compulsion to use a drug, loss of control over its use, and continued use despite adverse consequences. The model further holds that once individuals develop the disease of drug addiction, they can never return to social drug use. Abstinence is the only effective long-term treatment of the disease.

The disease model allows health professionals to use familiar techniques to make a diagnosis, develop a treatment plan, educate a patient, and discuss the prognosis. It obligates health professionals to address the problem in a nonjudgmental manner.

The American Medical Association, the American Psychiatric Association, and the World Health Organization consider alcoholism and other drug-addicted states to be a disease.

CONCLUSIONS

Drug abuse, which includes the abuse of alcohol, is common-place among teenagers and, to some extent, preteens as well. The consequences of children using drugs can be grave. Parents, teachers, and counselors should know the answers to the previously mentioned 15 questions about drug abuse which are presented in subsequent chapters and summarized in the Epilogue to this volume.

Many theories exist as to why some individuals become addicted to drugs while others do not. These theories can be summarized in four models—biological model, psychological model, social model, and disease model. The disease model is particularly helpful because it allows health professionals to use familiar techniques and obligates them to address the problem in a nonjudgmental manner.

2

What Are Drugs of Abuse?

Drugs of abuse are chemical substances that exert a mood-altering effect on the brain and which are capable of producing addiction. They are abused for the feelings they produce.

GENERIC NAMES VERSUS TRADE NAMES

Legal drugs are described by generic names and trade names. They are prescribed by physicians or sold over-the-counter. Many of them, especially some of the prescription drugs, are frequently abused. Generic names are related to the chemical structure of the drug. Every drug has a different chemical structure. Trade names, on the other hand, are names given to drugs by the pharmaceutical companies who manufacture them. When several companies manufacture the same drug, it will have more than one trade name.

Generic names traditionally begin with a lower case letter and trade names begin with an upper case letter. For example, propoxyphene (generic name) is called Darvon by one manufacturer and SK-65 by another one. Darvon and SK-65 are trade names. Trade names are often placed in parentheses behind the generic name; for example, propoxyphene (Darvon, SK-65).

Since illicit drugs are manufactured illegally, they do not have trade names. They do, however, have slang names. For example, in the drug culture, marijuana is known as grass, LSD as acid, and PCP as angel dust. They, like prescription drugs, have generic names. The generic name for the principle drug in marijuana is delta-9-THC, for LSD it is lysergic acid diethylamide, and for PCP it is phencyclidine.

CLASSIFICATION OF DRUGS BY THEIR EFFECTS ON THE BRAIN

Classification of drugs of abuse by this method is most helpful because all drugs in the same group have similar effects on the brain and produce similar withdrawal symptoms. Drugs of abuse are generally divided into eight groups: (1) depressants, (2) opioids, (3) stimulants, (4) cannabinoids, (5) phencyclidines, (6) inhalants, (7) anabolic steroids, and (8) hallucinogens.

1. *Depressants.* The depressant drugs depress excitable tissues in the brain. They decrease inhibitions, relieve anxiety, sedate, and intoxicate. This group of drugs includes alcohol, barbiturates (Amytal, Luminal, Seconal), barbiturate-like drugs (Doriden, Placidyl, Quaalude), meprobamate (Miltown, Equanil), benzo-diazepines (Valium, Librium, Xanax, Ativan, Halcion), and chloral hydrate (Noctec). Drugs in this class are known as *sedative-hypnotics. Sedatives* produce calm and relaxation. *Hypnotics* induce sleep.

2. *Opioids.* Opioids, known clinically as *narcotics*, are used to treat pain and to suppress cough and diarrhea. They also produce euphoria and sedation. They are classified as naturally occurring (opium, morphine, codeine), semisynthetic (heroin, Dilaudid, Percodan), and synthetic (Demerol, Darvon, Lomotil). A fourth group, the *agonist–antagonist* opioids (Talwin, Stadol, Nu-

bain), are also synthetic. This latter group is so named because these drugs possess properties of both narcotics (agonist effect) and drugs that block the effects of narcotics (antagonist effect).

3. *Stimulants.* Drugs in this group produce excitement and euphoria, decrease appetite, and decrease the need for sleep. The primary drugs in this group are cocaine, amphetamines (Dexedrine, Benzedrine, Desoxyn), and a group of diet pills (Tenuate, Preludin, Fastin). Nicotine is also a stimulant.

4. *Cannabinoids.* The cannabinoids (marijuana, hashish, hash oil) produce a sense of detachment, euphoria, and altered time sense.

5. *Phencyclidine.* There are at least 60 drugs related to phencyclidine (PCP). Phencyclidine, known in the drug culture as "angel dust," and its related compounds produce intoxication, muscle rigidity, and reduced pain perception.

6. *Inhalants.* The inhalants are volatile, liquid substances whose fumes are inhaled directly or are gases that are inhaled. They include solvents and aerosols (glues, gasoline, paint thinners, Liquid Paper, Scotchgard), nitrites (amyl nitrite, butyl nitrite), and nitrous oxide, which is used in the dental profession as an anesthetic ("laughing gas"). The inhalants produce altered states of consciousness, primarily light-headedness, euphoria, and confusion.

7. *Anabolic steroids.* Drugs in this group are related to the male sex hormone testosterone. They are abused primarily in attempts to increase muscle mass and athletic performance. They produce euphoria, decreased fatigue, and libido changes, and may also produce aggressive behavior. They include a group that is used orally (Anavar, Dianabol, Halotestin) and another group that is used intramuscularly (Durabolin, Delatestryl, DEPO-Testosterone).

8. *Hallucinogens.* Drugs in this group produce hallucinations—seeing, hearing, or smelling things that are not there. Hallucinogens include lysergic acid diethylamide (LSD), mescaline (peyote cactus), and psilocybin (mushrooms).

FEDERAL GOVERNMENT CLASSIFICATION

Another important classification of drugs of abuse is that of the Federal Comprehensive Drug Abuse Prevention and Control Act, passed by Congress in 1970 to regulate the manufacture, distribution, and dispensing of controlled substances. This act established five schedules of drugs, with varying degrees of control for each schedule. Drugs were placed in appropriate schedules based on three main criteria—potential for abuse, accepted medical use, and potential to produce dependence (addiction).

1. *Schedule I.* Drugs in this class have very high potentials for abuse and dependence and have no currently accepted medical uses. Drugs in Schedule I include heroin, LSD, and marijuana.

2. *Schedule II.* Drugs in this class have high potentials for abuse and dependence; however, they have currently accepted medical uses. Schedule II drugs include morphine, cocaine, and secobarbital (Seconal, a sleeping pill).

3. *Schedule III.* Drugs in this class have lower potentials for abuse and dependence than drugs in Schedule II, and they have currently accepted medical uses. Schedule III drugs include paregoric, benzphetamine (a diet pill), anabolic steroids (Halotestin, Dianabol, Durabolin), and combinations of aspirin or acetaminophen (Tylenol) with small doses of codeine.

4. *Schedule IV.* Drugs in this class have lower potentials for abuse and dependence than drugs in Schedule III. They also have currently accepted medical uses. Schedule IV drugs include diazepam (Valium), propoxyphene (Darvon), and pemoline (Cylert), which is a medication for hyperactive children.

5. *Schedule V.* Drugs in this class have very low potentials for abuse and dependence and have currently accepted medical uses. Schedule V drugs are mixtures containing limited quantities of narcotics and nonnarcotic ingredients. Examples are diphenoxylate plus atropine (Lomotil) for diarrhea and hydrocodone plus phenyltoloxamine (Tussionex) for cough.

CONCLUSIONS

Drugs of abuse are chemical substances that alter the way people feel and which are capable of producing addiction.

Prescription drugs are described by chemical or generic names and by names given to them by their manufacturer (trade names). Illicit drugs do not have trade names, but they do have generic names and slang or street names.

Drugs are classified into eight groups according to their effects on the brain. They are also classified into five groups by the Drug Enforcement Association according to their potential for abuse, accepted medical use, and potential to produce addiction.

3

How Do Drugs of Abuse Differ from Other Drugs?

CHARACTERISTICS OF DRUGS OF ABUSE

Drugs of abuse possess certain characteristics that other drugs do not:

- They produce an altered mood state such as sedation, relaxation, or euphoria.
- These effects reinforce the drug use; that is, the feelings aroused by the drug make the user want to use it again.
- Compulsive use occurs; the user feels as though he must have the drug.
- Use continues despite the known, harmful effects. Many alcoholics, for example, continue to drink despite severe, irreversible liver damage.
- Regular and temporal patterns of use occur. Drug users tend to use drugs on a regular basis and at specific times during the day. One patient, for example, broke out in a cold sweat, felt anxious, and developed a rapid heart rate at six o'clock every evening. The problem was quite obviously not withdrawal because it had been far too long since her last cocaine use. The mystery was solved when it was discov-

ered that her usual pattern was to use cocaine at six o'clock every evening when she arrived home from work. She was experiencing an intense craving for the drug.

- Deprivation increases the desire to use the drug. A good example of this is the rush to the lobby during the intermission of a play by cigarette smokers.
- Paired stimuli increases use. The sight of a cocaine pipe on a television program can stimulate an intense craving for cocaine in a recovering cocaine addict.
- Tolerance develops. With regular use of a drug, more and more of the drug becomes required to produce the same effects. Nonaddicting drugs do not possess this property.
- Physical dependence may develop; that is, regular, prolonged use of a drug may produce withdrawal symptoms on cessation of use.
- The relapse rate is high. Many drug users quit several times before finally achieving permanent abstinence.

ABSTINENCE SYNDROMES

Withdrawal symptoms sometimes occur when individuals stop using drugs. Each drug group has its own set of withdrawal symptoms, known as an *abstinence syndrome*. The severity of abstinence syndromes ranges from that of the depressant drugs, which may be life-threatening, to a complete lack of an abstinence syndrome as with the hallucinogenic drugs.

Drug group	Severity of abstinence syndrome
Depressants	++++
Opioids	+++
Stimulants	++
Cannabinoids	++
Phencyclidines	++
Inhalants	+
Anabolic steroids	+
Hallucinogens	−

The most severe withdrawal, delirium tremens from alcohol, sometimes results in death, even with good medical care.

The major withdrawal symptoms usually run their course five days after stopping the use of most drugs; however, minor symptoms, called *postacute abstinence syndrome*, may last for weeks to months. Severe abstinence syndromes usually do not occur in adolescents.

HOW DRUGS AFFECT THE BRAIN

To understand how drugs exert their influences on the brain, it is first necessary to understand the function of the limbic system; how *neurons* (nerve cells) transmit information from one site in the body to another, and how the *synapse* (junction between neurons) functions.

The Limbic System

All drugs of abuse act in the brain to change the way one feels, which is why they are called *psychoactive substances*. It is the feelings produced by drugs that users seek. People, then, get addicted to feelings, not drugs. The cocaine addict, for example, would be just as happy getting the "high" from the stimulation of an electrode placed in the pleasure center of his brain as from doses of cocaine.

The part of the brain that is responsible for feelings is called the *limbic system*. This is where drugs of abuse produce their effects. The limbic system is located deep within the brain. The hypothalamus, which contains the pleasure center of the brain, is part of the limbic system.

Drugs, as we will see, produce feelings by altering the functioning of natural biochemicals in the limbic system, called *neurotransmitters*.

The Neuron

Neurons are the transmission lines of the nervous system. A pinprick to the big toe, for example, initiates electrical impulses, or *action potentials,* in local nerve endings. These impulses then travel up a series of three neurons, crossing two synapses, to reach the brain where they are sensed as pain. Neurons also transmit information from one site in the brain to another.

The Synapse

Drugs exert their effects primarily by altering the functioning of synapses in the brain. To understand the effects of drugs, it is necessary, therefore, to understand the synapse and how it normally functions (Fig. 3.1). As action potentials move along the presynaptic neuron, they reach the nerve terminal where they act on storage vesicles to cause the release of specific neurotransmitter molecules. The neurotransmitter molecules then cross the synaptic cleft—a space between neurons—where they briefly interact with receptors on the postsynaptic neuron. This interaction produces secondary action potentials which then continue the signal

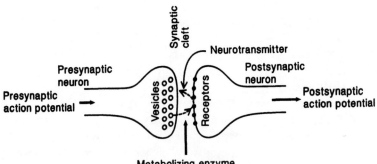

Figure 3.1. The synapse. (From H. T. Milhorn, Jr., *Chemical Dependence: Diagnosis, Treatment, and Prevention,* Springer-Verlag, New York, 1990. Reprinted with permission.)

on its route. After the brief interaction with the receptors, the neurotransmitter molecules tend to return to the presynaptic vesicles for storage and reuse. However, a portion of the neurotransmitter molecules are inactivated by an enzyme in the synaptic cleft. Synaptic transmission is extremely rapid, requiring only about 1/1000 of a second.

How Drugs Alter Synaptic Function

Drugs alter synaptic function by a variety of mechanisms:

- Administration of substances that are converted by the body into the neurotransmitters increases the availability of the neurotransmitter in the presynaptic storage vesicles. This, in turn, causes an excess release of neurotransmitter molecules in response to incoming action potentials, thereby increasing synaptic cleft neurotransmitter concentration. This makes more neurotransmitter molecules available for stimulation of the postsynaptic receptors, resulting in enhanced signal transmission across the synapse.
- Some drugs decrease the activity of the metabolizing enzyme, thereby increasing the synaptic cleft neurotransmitter concentration and, hence, synaptic transmission.
- Other drugs mimic the activity of the neurotransmitter itself on the postsynaptic receptors and increase synaptic transmission in this manner.
- Some drugs block access of the neurotransmitter molecules to the postsynaptic receptors, thereby reducing signal transmission across the synapse.
- Other drugs block the reuptake of the neurotransmitter by the presynaptic storage vesicles, thus increasing the neurotransmitter concentration in the synaptic cleft and, hence, synaptic transmission.
- Some drugs stimulate the release of neurotransmitter molecules from the presynaptic storage vesicles, increasing synaptic cleft neurotransmitter concentration and, hence, synaptic transmission.

If the synapses affected by a specific drug happen to be located in the pleasure center of the brain, enhanced transmission of the signal is sensed as euphoria (pleasure), and decreased transmission as dysphoria (depression).

The Neurotransmitters

Six neurotransmitters—gamma-aminobutyric acid, acetylcholine, norepinephrine, dopamine, serotonin, and beta-endorphin—account for most of the effects produced by the action of drugs of abuse on the brain.

Gamma-aminobutyric acid (GABA)

Unlike other neurotransmitters, GABA acts in the brain to inhibit synaptic transmission. Drugs that exert their effects through the GABA neurotransmitter system include all of the depressants. Phencyclidine (PCP) has an effect on all six neurotransmitters, including GABA.

Acetylcholine

This neurotransmitter counterbalances the effects of dopamine (see below) and functions in initiating short-term memory as well as maintaining memory. Phencyclidine and nicotine influence the acetylcholine neurotransmitter system.

Norepinephrine

This neurotransmitter is responsible for modulating mood and maintaining sleep states. It is affected primarily by the stimulant drugs and also by phencyclidine and the opioid or narcotic drugs.

Dopamine

This neurotransmitter serves to counterbalance the effects of acetylcholine. In addition, it stimulates the pleasure center, modulates mood, affects intellectual processes, and inhibits prolactin release. Prolactin is a hormone involved in milk production in nursing mothers. Dopamine is affected by the stimulant drugs, as well as phencyclidine.

Serotonin

This neurotransmitter is involved in modulating mood, initiating sleep, and rapid eye movement (REM) sleep, which is the portion of sleep in which dreams occur. It is affected by the hallucinogenic group of drugs and phencyclidine.

Beta-endorphin

This neurotransmitter is involved in modulating mood and in pain perception. It also inhibits norepinephrine release. It is affected by the opioid group of drugs, as well as phencyclidine.

The neurotransmitters responsible for the effects of marijuana and anabolic steroids have not yet been identified.

THE PRIMITIVE SURVIVAL BRAIN CONCEPT

The primitive survival brain concept of drug addiction is based on the premise that millions of years ago on the evolutionary tree, humans did not possess a reasoning, thinking brain—the cerebral cortex—but instead depended entirely on a rudimentary brain whose single purpose was survival. This primitive brain served to find food and water, flee or fight when circumstances dictated, and have sex for survival of the species. The limbic system is part of this primitive brain. As time passed, the cerebral cortex evolved around the primitive brain.

Drug addiction is considered to involve movement of control from the cerebral cortex to the primitive brain (Fig. 3.2). In the use stage, the message from the cerebral cortex is, "I think I'll use some cocaine." Using cocaine is a matter of choice. Once the dopamine system in the old survival brain is sufficiently deranged from chronic cocaine use to signal addiction, the cerebral cortex loses control to the primitive survival brain which now sends the message, "If I don't get some cocaine, I'm going to die." Getting the cocaine has become a matter of survival. The wall has been crossed. This explains why addicted individuals will lie, cheat, steal, and prostitute to get drugs when they otherwise would not do so.

DENIAL

Denial is most simply defined as not recognizing a problem, even in the face of significant adverse consequences and despite the fact that the problem is evident to others. Denial is not lying. It

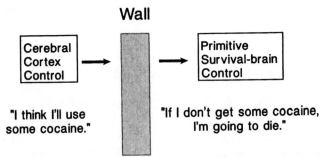

Figure 3.2. The primitive survival-brain concept of chemical dependence. (From H. T. Milhorn, Jr., *Chemical Dependence: Diagnosis, Treatment, and Prevention*, Springer-Verlag, New York, 1990. Reprinted with permission.)

occurs, for the most part, at a subconscious level. It is the major symptom of addiction.

Mechanism of Denial

In the use stage, drugs act on the limbic system to produce a drug craving (Fig. 3.3). The drug craving then causes the cerebral cortex to produce what I call addictive behaviors; that is, the lying, stealing, and cheating that take place to get the drugs. These behaviors then produce guilt, which normally serves to reduce or eliminate the drug use as shown by the broken line. Once addiction develops, however, the adolescent is unable to moderate his or her addictive behaviors because of the overwhelming drug craving produced by the limbic system. The behaviors, therefore, continue despite the intense guilt. To protect the mind from the psychological pain produced by this internal conflict between drug use and guilt, denial develops as a way of relieving the guilt. The relationship between the drug use and its effects is not clearly seen by the addict. Drug use is bad behavior. Drug addiction is the disease.

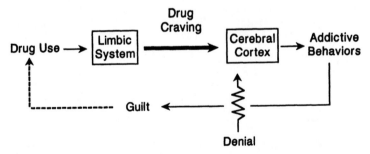

Figure 3.3. Mechanism of denial. (From H. T. Milhorn, Jr., *Chemical Dependence: Diagnosis, Treatment, and Prevention*, Springer-Verlag, New York, 1990. Reprinted with permission.)

Denial is not unique to drug addicts. It occurs in other circumstances as well. For example, it is the first stage in the grief process—denial → anger → bargaining → depression → acceptance. Following the sudden death of one's spouse or child, for instance, denial immediately sets in to protect the mind from the overwhelming grief that would otherwise occur.

Tools for Achieving Denial

Denial serves to perpetuate drug addiction, sometimes for years. Drug-addicted adolescents use at least eight tools to achieve denial:

1. *Rationalization.* Using socially acceptable but untrue explanations for inappropriate behavior: "I have to take more narcotics than prescribed because my headaches are so bad."

2. *Projection.* Blaming others for one's own failings and inadequacies: "I wouldn't have to drink so much if my parents would just leave me alone."

3. *Minimization.* Underestimating the magnitude of their drug use.

4. *Repression.* Unconsciously excluding from one's conscious mind unbearable thoughts, feelings, or experiences.

5. *Suppression.* Consciously excluding from one's conscious mind unbearable thoughts, feelings, or experiences.

6. *Isolation.* Avoiding relationships that might interfere with their drug use.

7. *Regression.* Reverting to a level of emotional maturity appropriate to an earlier stage in life.

8. *Conversion.* Expressing emotional conflicts through physical symptoms. Conversion allows addicts to focus on minor physical problems so as to avoid dealing with their drug addiction.

Denial can take a number of forms: (1) "My problems are not due to drug abuse," (2) "Drugs cause adverse consequences in others, not me," and (3) "Some drugs, or ways of using drugs, are okay. Others are not." The first two forms of denial are relatively straightforward and easy to recognize. The third form, however, can be subtle. Consider the following illustration: I had a patient who regularly abused Luminal, a barbiturate, by intravenous injection. He switched to Librium (a benzodiazepine) when Luminal temporarily became unavailable. The contents of the Librium capsules did not dissolve very readily, so that when he accidentally injected the material into an artery instead of the vein, it plugged up the small blood vessels in the distal part of his arm, causing bloodflow to stop. This led to surgical amputation of his arm just below the shoulder. From his point of view, the mistake was not that he had used drugs intravenously but that he had switched to Librium. Intravenous drug use according to him is okay as long as you are careful about which drugs you use. This form of denial served a purpose for him. It kept the door open for future use of intravenous Luminal. After all, to his way of thinking his drug of choice was not what caused him to lose the arm.

CONCLUSIONS

Drugs of abuse possess a number of characteristics that nonaddicting drugs do not. Among these, withdrawal symptoms sometimes occur when adolescents stop using drugs.

Drugs of abuse produce their effects by altering chemicals in the brain known as neurotransmitters. This alteration causes a change in the way people feel, usually producing pleasure.

Denial, the principal symptom of drug addiction, functions to perpetuate the addiction. For the most part, denial occurs at a subconscious level. It serves to protect the mind from the psychological pain which would otherwise be produced by the internal conflict between drug abuse and guilt.

4

Is Alcoholism Truly a Disease?

Over the past several years, there has been considerable debate among the lay public about whether or not alcoholism is truly a disease, as opposed to a lack of willpower, a bad habit, or immoral behavior. What evidence do we have that alcoholism is actually a disease?

RESEARCH STUDIES

The important association between alcoholic individuals and a history of alcoholism in their families was first noted over 50 years ago. Since then it has been shown that the risk of becoming alcoholic and possibly the severity of the alcoholism directly relates to the closeness of the genetic relationship to alcoholic family members.

Given the above relationship, the obvious question then becomes, "Is the increased risk of alcoholism genetically determined or is it a learned condition from having grown up in an alcoholic family?" A number of studies have been conducted to answer this question.

Early support for the genetic factor began to appear as early as 1949 when it was discovered that some rats, when deprived of vitamin B complex, developed a craving for alcohol. When these animals were bred, seven generations later their offspring also preferred alcohol over water.

In 1969, an animal model of alcoholism was developed through selective breeding. One strain of black mice loved alcohol; another strain hated it. Using these two strains of mice, scientists were able to demonstrate differences in brain chemistry, particularly in the reward areas of the brain.

In 1979, Goodwin found that children of alcoholics had the same rate of alcoholism regardless of whether they were brought up in their parents' homes or adopted at early ages into nonalcoholic homes. Shortly afterwards, scientists studying over 5000 adoptees in Denmark found that sons of alcoholics adopted by other families were almost four times as likely to become alcoholic as the adopted sons of nonalcoholics. Similar results were found in a separate study in Sweden.

Twin studies were pursued to better separate out the relative importance of genetic versus environmental factors. These studies are based on the fact that there are two types of twins. Identical twins share 100 percent of their genes while nonidentical twins share only 50 percent of their genes. Thus, if alcoholism were related to genetic factors, the risk for the disorder should be significantly higher in the identical twin of an alcoholic than the nonidentical twin of an alcoholic. This assumption proved to be true.

In 1990, Blum *et al.* attempted to identify the gene responsible for transmission of the hereditary tendency to become alcoholic. When comparing the genetic make-up of deceased alcoholics with that of nonalcoholics, they found that 69 percent of the alcoholics had a particular gene form (dopamine D_2 receptor, A_1 allele), whereas 80 percent of the nonalcoholics lacked it. They postulated from this that individuals with this particular gene are at higher risk of becoming alcoholic than those without it.

THE NATURAL COURSE OF ALCOHOLISM

Every illness, if left untreated, follows a natural course or progression. Jellinek has shown that the natural course of alcoholism, for most alcoholics, can be divided into six stages: (1) the prealcoholism stage, (2) the early alcoholism stage, (3) the acute stage, (4) the early chronic stage, (5) the late chronic stage, and (6) death. There is no time limit for the entire course or for any of its stages. Some alcoholics progress more slowly through the stages than others. In some, progression through some stages is prolonged while progression through others is very brief. For the most part, from the time an individual begins to lose control to the time when he or she passes into the final stages of alcoholism requires, on the average, fifteen years for men and seven to eight years for women. The reason for this difference is not known. As an example, let us follow the progression of alcoholism in a typical alcoholic. For the sake of discussion, we will consider the alcoholic to be male.

Prealcoholism Stage

The prealcoholism stage covers all of an individual's drinking history from the time of his first drink until just prior to showing the symptoms of alcoholism. Throughout this stage there is a gradual increase in drinking, both in frequency of drinking and in the quantity of alcohol consumed. Usually, the individual is unaware of the fact that he finds more and more occasions for drinking. He finds in alcohol a relief from tensions and, while drinking, experiences feelings of freedom, adequacy, and confidence which he may not usually have. What was once occasional relief drinking becomes regular relief drinking in this stage. A gradual increase in tolerance also occurs. Solitary drinking rarely occurs in this stage, although it may begin.

Early Alcoholism Stage

In this stage the symptoms of alcoholism begin to appear.

1. *Blackouts*. This is usually the first symptom of alcoholism to appear. Typically, the individual has three to four drinks at a

party, and there may be only a little obvious change in his behavior. The next day, however, he remembers nothing about what went on the evening before.

2. *Sneaks drinks.* Drinking now means more to him than it does to most average drinkers. Not wanting his friends or family to know how much he drinks, he tends to drink on the sly. At a party or other social function, he takes as many refills as he can without appearing too obvious. If he finds himself in a situation where it is especially difficult to get enough to drink, he may even finish someone else's partially consumed drink.

3. *Drinking before parties and social gatherings.* Drinking too much on occasion at a party is apt to be overlooked as something that could happen to anyone, but arriving in an intoxicated state is often looked upon as a different matter. If alcoholic beverages are not being served, his drinking may be resented even more. This resentment may result in him being left out of future parties, marking the beginning of his gradual isolation from close friends, long-standing business relationships, and social relationships.

4. *Gulping drinks.* Leisurely consumption no longer is satisfactory because it does not bring an immediate reward. As a result, he has a tendency to gulp the first two or three drinks prior to settling into the more socially approved practice of sipping.

5. *Avoids talking about drinking.* Realizing that he drinks too much, he begins to experience feelings of guilt and embarrassment. He avoids talking about drinking for fear that his drinking will be brought into the conversation. Whenever drinking does come up, he makes every effort to change the subject.

6. *Blackouts become more frequent.* More and more, blackouts cause concern because they increasingly create problems in his social, business, and domestic life. For example, he may stop in a tavern for a few drinks on the way to a business appointment. The next day he may be extremely upset because he had too much to drink and missed the appointment. After calling to apologize and offer an excuse, he discovers that he kept his appointment; however, he remembers nothing of the business transacted. Similar and repeated experiences of this nature in the business and social

world soon gives him a reputation of unreliability and puts him further along the way to isolation.

7. *Rarely gets drunk before evening.* Up to this point, the alcoholic rarely becomes intoxicated before the evening. When he is through with his work he is eager to get home so he can start drinking. His drinking is progressively becoming more of a problem. He occasionally calls in to work "sick" because of a morning hangover.

Acute Stage

The acute stage is marked by a worsening of the previous symptoms and the introduction of new ones. The conflicting emotions of the alcoholic result in personal frustration and unreasonable behavior.

1. *Winds up drunk.* In this stage, the alcoholic first experiences loss of control over his drinking. For example, with 15 minutes on his hands before a business appointment, he may slip into a bar to have a couple of drinks. Two to three hours later he staggers out, having had a dozen or more. He didn't intend to get drunk. He certainly didn't mean to miss his appointment, but once he began drinking he was unable to stop until he was intoxicated. These episodes increase with frequency as he moves on into the acute stage. Inwardly, he is concerned about them but becomes incensed if anyone mentions the problem to him.

Despite his problems, he does not believe that he will never be able to regain control over his drinking. In fact, he sets out on a long, futile and frustrating campaign to demonstrate to the world that he can drink like other people. Each time he begins to drink, he is convinced that this time he will be able to stop at only one or two drinks.

2. *Solitary drinking.* If solitary drinking began in the early alcoholism stage as it occasionally does, it now becomes a regular pattern. Rather than going to a tavern to do his drinking, he goes

to a place of seclusion such as a hotel, motel, or his own home and remains in a state of intoxication from a day or two to a week or more. Thus, he becomes more and more isolated, a process that will be repeated many times with increasing frequency. These episodes leave him embarrassed and ashamed.

3. *Rationalization.* The alcoholic has an overwhelming sense of guilt because of his excessive drinking and resulting unreasonable behavior; however, he quickly learns to rationalize that it is not his fault. It is because his wife nagged him, his boss bawled him out, or a friend crossed him. If it were not for the unreasonable attitudes of others, he reasons, he would have no trouble whatsoever controlling his drinking. He begins to feel that rules which apply to others do not apply to him and that he should be accorded privileges not granted to others. These rationalizations progressively become more and more unreasonable.

4. *Loss of self-esteem.* Even though he may refuse to make any open admissions that his drinking is creating serious problems, he is forced to make this admission to himself. His self-esteem diminishes to the point where he finds it necessary to constantly devise ways of bolstering his ego.

5. *Extravagant behavior.* At times, he attempts to revive his waning self-esteem. He may buy his wife or family an expensive gift that is impractical, useless, or beyond their financial means. For example, he may purchase his wife a fur coat which cannot be worn because of her shabby and depleted wardrobe. There are other things that transiently give him the feeling that he can compel the world to reckon with his power. Little things, such as giving a big tip, riding in a taxi, or making a long distance phone call make him feel like a big shot. This is known as *grandiosity*.

When he is sober he senses what harm he is doing to his family and friends and so, bolstered by a drink or two, sets about to deprive himself of things he wants to make up for what he has caused them to suffer.

6. *Becomes aggressive.* As criticism increases, he develops an inner anger which eventually breaks forth as aggression, usually directed at someone or something remote from the person against

whom he harbors ill will. For example, he may kick in a window at home because his boss made him angry.

7. *Experiences remorse.* His nasty disposition and aggressive behavior further complicate his life through brushes with the law and increased strained relationships with friends and family. It seems to him that no matter what he does everything turns out wrong. Before he can set his life straight, another drinking bout gets in the way. He continually asks himself, "Why me? Why can't I drink like other people?" Finally, it dawns on him that it really isn't him: The world has dealt him a bum deal despite the fact that he has "done his best."

8. *Periodic abstinence.* Even though his drinking is increasing and his bouts of drunkenness are more frequent, he still has his periods of sobriety when, for a time, he seems to be almost his normal self again. During these times, he is better able to reason out his problems and comes to the conclusion that he will have to give up drinking—not for good, just until he can be sure that he has at last regained control of it. These periods of sobriety last a few days, a few weeks, or several months, and serve the purpose of demonstrating to his friends and to his family, but most importantly to him, that he can take alcohol or leave it. Eventually, he feels that it is safe for him to drink again, and so he does. Remorsefully, sobering up he is convinced that the next time will be different. Of course, it and subsequent alcoholic bouts are not.

9. *Changes drinking pattern.* During one of his sober periods, when he is reviewing his problem yet again, he suddenly comes to believe that he has found the answer. It isn't him. It isn't drinking. He just hasn't been going about it right. The real secret is to drink the right kind of alcoholic beverage, to drink only at certain times and at certain places, and to drink only with certain people. He puts his plan into action, and for a time it seems to work. But with increased self-confidence comes lessened discretion in carrying out the plan. Ultimately, he awakens from a drunken binge with characteristic familiarity.

10. *Walks out on friends and employers.* He broods over his latest failed plan and is certain that his family and friends view it with

an "I told you so" attitude. He reasons that they never give him any credit—they don't understand. They don't even try. He comes to feel it just isn't worth it. When the opportunity arises, he walks out on his friends and tells off the boss or quits before he can be fired.

Early Chronic Stage

In the early chronic stage, the complete exhaustion of the alcoholic's alibis and rationalizations is matched by the physical and mental deterioration arising out of long abuse of body and mind.

Drinking takes on a major importance, and the alcoholic undergoes a marked change in attitude. Previously, he evidenced genuine concern about his drinking interfering with his activities and responsibilities, whereas he now becomes increasingly concerned about his activities and responsibilities interfering with his drinking. His attitude changes to one of abandon, indifference, and unconcern. Friendship is no longer determined by the standards that were once so important to him. A chance acquaintance, after only a few drinks, can rapidly qualify as a confidant for the most sacred concerns of his heart. Drinking has become more important than anything else in the world and nothing must be allowed to interfere with it. His former interests—church, clubs, lodges, etc.—are forgotten.

1. *Family life changes.* It is inevitable that with his complete preoccupation with alcohol and increasing disregard for family interests, family members should retaliate with decreased interest in his welfare. Diminishing attention to him at home only serves to strengthen his anger and confirm his belief that no one really understands or cares about him.

2. *Experiences great self-pity.* His pity turns inward and is lavished generously on himself. He focuses on the injustices he feels have been done to him by just about everybody he can think

of. He sees himself as a paragon of virtue, patience, and unselfishness, and as one who has gone far out of his way, without regard
for his personal inconvenience, to serve the interest of others; but
to no avail. His efforts and consideration on behalf of others have
never been appreciated. It's no wonder he took to drinking too
much.

3. *Attempts geographic cure.* He reasons that he is not to blame
for his troubles. Instead, it is the fault of the community, his
family, and his job. He is not appreciated here. He hasn't been
given a chance. The thing to do is to escape, to go where he is not
known and start a brand new life; then he will be able to control his
drinking. He may move to a new location, another city or another
state. He may, in fact, stay sober for a few days, find a job, and
appear to have found a solution to his problem. But before long he
begins to feel lonely. The only place he is certain of finding
understanding fellowship is in a bar or tavern, so he sets out to
have a few drinks. Several days later, when he sobers up, he
remembers telling his new boss that he wasn't a drinking man—
maybe just a nip now and then. Thus, he sets off again to make a
new start and build a new life.

4. *Hospitalization.* The cumulative effects of heavy drinking
and poor health habits are becoming evident. He begins to develop alcohol-related disorders such as cirrhosis of the liver, pancreatitis, and peptic ulcer disease. At this point, hospitalization for
one or more of these ailments takes place, usually following a
particularly severe and prolonged drinking bout. His unpleasant
hospital experience leads to two basic fears: (1) that someday he
may be deprived of alcohol again, and (2) that alcohol itself will let
him down, and will no longer provide him the satisfaction and
relief he has come to expect. The first fear leads him to hoarding as
much liquor as he can. He hides it in the closet, in the back of the
bottom drawer in a cabinet, in the garage, and in his car—a
phenomenon known as *guarding your supply.* The second fear is
one he can do nothing about. It lingers and torments him in the
days to come.

5. *Decrease in sexual energy.* To further complicate his mental

frustration, he experiences a rather marked decrease in sex drive. This serves to increase his hostility toward his girlfriend or wife, while he rationalizes that the problem is with her, not him. He becomes convinced that she must be having extramarital relations with other men. Nothing will convince him otherwise. This phenomenon gives rise to the term *alcoholic jealousy*.

6. *Morning drinking*. His suspicion, fear, resentment, frustration, and remorse continue to increase his need for alcohol. For some time he has been drinking on the sly, catching a few quick ones during the day. If circumstances of his job do not allow this to be done openly, he may sneak in something to drink in his lunch pail or even stash away small bottles, enough for a nip or two, in his pockets. As his problems grow beyond his ability to cope with them for even a few hours, he develops the habit of drinking regularly in the morning. He feels that he has to have an "eye opener" to get him started for the day.

Late Chronic Stage

In this stage of the alcoholic's life, he experiences total social isolation from normal people and circumstances as well as gross physical deterioration, with marked susceptibility to disease and ever increasing mental confusion. His ability to hold a job is markedly impaired, and he is no longer able to hide his drinking.

1. *Prolonged benders*. With his drinking now a matter of common knowledge in the community, he no longer hides it. He goes on prolonged benders during which time he shows a complete lack of responsibility toward any of his normal obligations. At the same time, he shows a marked deterioration in ethical standards, showing almost no regard for the rights, wishes, or feelings of others. His every thought and action is selfishly concerned with what he can do for his own comfort and convenience. In addition, he begins to experience difficulty in thinking. He has trouble remembering little things in their proper relationships and, at times, is unable to reason through matters of the simplest nature.

2. *Loss of morale.* He begins to turn to people far below his station in life. Anyone who offers him a drink is his "buddy," and he is seemingly indifferent to how crude, vulgar, or uncouth they are. He is rapidly becoming just as crude, vulgar, and uncouth.

3. *Drinks nonbeverage alcohol.* Life is becoming increasingly more unbearable, and jobs are becoming more difficult to obtain. He only sobers up when he runs out of money. If he is in a real financial bind and his craving is particularly intense, he drinks anything he can get—rubbing alcohol, canned heat (Sterno), or vanilla extract.

4. *Decrease in tolerance.* Up to this point, achieving his desired state of intoxication has required him to drink more and more alcohol. Now, probably due to his deteriorating liver, he finds that it requires less to induce stupor than it once did, a condition known as *reverse tolerance.*

5. *Unnamed fears.* Daylight has become a time of fear because he feels naked and transparent before the world. He feels as if his life is an open book for everyone to read. Night is no better, since darkness causes him to feel the bitter desolation of his life.

6. *Tremors.* He begins to have tremors. His hands shake and his lips quiver. The closer to being sober he becomes, the worse the tremors get. Eventually, he gets to the point where he is even unable to tie his shoelaces, button his shirt, or wind his watch until he has first had a few drinks to steady his hands.

7. *Drinking to relieve the symptoms of drinking.* He is now drinking to relieve the symptoms brought on by too many years of persistent and excessive alcohol consumption which are, in turn, only temporarily relieved by more drinking.

8. *Interest in religion.* He looks around and sees in others fulfillment of ideals that once were his. Why did it have to happen to him? Others drink, but are able to control it. What's the difference between himself and them? He reasons that it must be because they are religious, or have undergone some religious experiences that he has never tried. Becoming even more desperate, he prays, a frantic calling out to God or anyone else who will

hear his calls for help. He feels as if he is going to go mad if something isn't done.

9. *Indifferent resignation.* Finally, for the first time in his life he admits that he is licked and assumes an attitude of indifferent resignation. He becomes embittered and resistant to any effort to change his way of life.

Death

Constant drunkenness has progressively taken its toll on his physical stamina and mental stability. Death finally occurs from suicide, from an accident, or from his severe alcohol-related health problems.

COMPARISON TO A KNOWN DISEASE

In medicine, we feel comfortable with the concept of a condition being a disease when we know several things about it: its etiology, its signs and symptoms, its natural course, its outcome if untreated, and whether a cure or treatment is available.

Since no one would argue against diabetes being a disease, let's compare this disorder to alcoholism.

Comparisons of Diabetes and Alcoholism

Etiology

• *Diabetes.* Diabetes runs in families. If a parent is diabetic, the children are at increased risk of developing the condition. Thus, there is a genetic component of the disease. However, since it is possible to develop diabetes without having it run in your family, other factors must also be involved.

• *Alcoholism.* As we have seen, alcoholism also runs in families. Studies of the genetics of this disorder leave little doubt that, for many, the tendency to become alcoholic is genetically transmitted from parents to children. Like diabetes, however, it is possible to become alcoholic without a family history, so that other factors must be involved as well.

Signs and Symptoms

• *Diabetes.* Signs and symptoms of diabetes include sugar in the urine, frequent urination, thirst, and fatigue.

• *Alcoholism.* Signs and symptoms of alcoholism, as we have seen, include blackouts, gulping the first few drinks, loss of control, guarding the supply, and continuing to drink despite adverse consequences.

Natural Course

• *Diabetes.* The natural course of untreated diabetes is, for both the condition and the adverse health problems that result from it, to become progressively worse.

• *Alcoholism.* The natural course of alcoholism, as we have seen, is also progressively downhill.

Untreated Outcome

• *Diabetes.* The ultimate outcome of untreated diabetes is death from its complications.

• *Alcoholism.* The ultimate outcome of untreated alcoholism, as we have seen, is also death.

Cure

• *Diabetes.* There is no known cure for diabetes.

• *Alcoholism.* There is no known cure for alcoholism.

Treatment

• *Diabetes.* Treatment of diabetes consists of medication such as insulin or pills, exercise, and diet.

• *Alcoholism.* Treatment of alcoholism consists primarily of behavior modification.

CONCLUSIONS

The current attitudes regarding alcoholism and other drug addictions, which view these as weaknesses, moral or ethical problems, bad habits, or a lack of willpower, are beginning to disappear as more of the facts become known.

Leprosy, epilepsy, and mental illness have all suffered from similar cultural prejudices in the past. Lepers were made to wear cowbells so they could be shunned, mentally ill patients were placed in chains or hidden away, and epileptics were burned at the stake because they were believed to be possessed by the devil. The pattern appears to be that first they are shunned; the clergy then castigate their morality; laws are then passed and legal sanctions invoked against them; they are then ignored by society; and finally, they are accepted as having a disease. Alcoholism seems to be following a similar pattern.

Scientific research clearly points to alcoholism as a disease, with a genetic transmission of the tendency to develop it. Alcoholism compares favorably to diabetes and other chronic diseases in terms of its characteristic etiology, signs and symptoms, natural course, untreated outcome, cure, and treatment. Based on existing evidence, the American Medical Association, the American Psychiatric Association, and the World Health Organization consider alcoholism and other drug dependencies to be a disease. So should we.

5

Why Do Adolescents Abuse Drugs?

THE NORMAL ADOLESCENT

Adolescence is defined as the period between the ages of 13 and 18. During this time, physical and psychological growth undergo significant development, and hormonal changes accelerate sexual maturation. As a result of these rapidly changing states, adolescents tend to feel awkward and insecure. They feel inadequate about their appearance and popularity. Adolescence for many is a time of frustration, anger, and rebellion.

Peer affiliation and desire for peer acceptance are hallmarks of adolescence. They feel the need for acceptance, praise, and approval by their peers more profoundly than in any other stage of life. Adolescents test limits and manipulate others. They tend to experiment with extremes of values and behaviors, and are often confused and scared. One minute they demand total independence, and the next they cry out for protection from themselves and the world in which they live. They often experience free-floating anxiety and identity crises, and commonly act out, which is a subconscious mechanism of expressing unacknowledged internal conflict. Adolescence is a period of exploration. Risk-taking and sensation-seeking behaviors are normal. Experimenting with drugs is now also a part of the adolescent's world.

THE DRUG ABUSE PROBLEM

Data on drug use by junior high school students and high school seniors from a nationwide study supported by the National Institute of Drug Abuse (Table 5.1) illustrate the extent of the problem among adolescents in the United States.

In addition to these data, 91 percent of high school seniors report having used alcohol at least once and 5 percent report using it daily.

More than two-thirds of high school seniors have smoked cigarettes at some time and 20 percent smoke them daily. The use of smokeless tobacco is increasing among adolescent boys. Twenty-two percent of 8th graders report using smokeless tobacco at some time in their lives, and 6.9 percent report using it in the

Table 5.1
Percent of Students Who Use Drugs
for 6th–8th Grades (JRHS) and 12th Grade *

	Annual use		Monthly use	
	JRHS	12th grade	JRHS	12th grade
Alcohol	41.0	73.3	14.9	44.7
Cigarettes	25.5	42.0	13.3	29.9
Marijuana	5.8	25.0	3.3	14.6
Cocaine	1.6	4.5	1.1	2.8
Other stimulants	3.0	9.3	1.8	5.0
Downers	2.2	5.3	1.4	3.4
Inhalants	4.8	5.1	2.3	2.7
Hallucinogens	1.9	8.0	1.2	3.8

*From the 1992–93 PRIDE survey of 236,745 students.

last month. However, only 0.2% percent of 8th graders report using it daily. The percentage of adolescents who use smokeless tobacco on a daily basis rises rapidly with increasing grade levels in high school.

Of high school seniors in a recent study, 65 percent report having used an illegal drug at least once, and 30 percent report having used an illegal drug prior to high school.

Data on high school seniors are somewhat conservative because students who drop out of school prior to their senior year are not included. Drug use among this group would be expected to be higher than among their in-school peers.

WHY ADOLESCENTS USE DRUGS

General Reasons

No simple answer exists to the perplexing question of why adolescents use alcohol and other drugs. Beyond the 5th grade, peers play the major role in shaping children's attitudes about drug use. Prior to this time, television and movies play the most influential role. The attitudes of parents toward alcohol and other drugs correlate strongly with the subsequent attitudes of their children.

Reasons Adolescents Give

Mackenzie and Jacobs have identified several reasons that adolescents give for using drugs. They use them:

As recreation	To conform
As a rite of passage	To prove sexuality
As a socializer	To reduce stress
For a new experience	To relieve anxiety

For pleasure	To relieve depression
In rebellion	To relieve fatigue
In response to an impulse	To relieve boredom
In self-exploration	To solve personal problems

However, the overwhelmingly predominant reason adolescents give for using drugs is that drugs make them feel good and they do not feel that they suffer adverse consequences from their use. They simply don't believe adults who tell them otherwise. Their peers confirm to them on a daily basis that their way of thinking is the correct one.

THE DRUG-ADDICTED ADOLESCENT

Differences from Adult Drug Addiction

Drug addiction in adolescents differs in several ways from that of adults. Adolescents lack adult coping skills, and most have not yet separated completely from their parents. Unlike adults, they are in the process of developing physically and psychologically. Drug abuse interferes with their psychological development.

Many adolescents feel sexually insecure and, in fact, may not have yet had their first sexual experience, although drug-abusing adolescents in general tend to be sexually promiscuous. Many have not yet experienced meaningful, loving, bonding relationships. Most still live at home and are not responsible for their financial support or for the financial support of others. Parents seldom withdraw food and shelter, so adolescents do not suffer the same consequences as adults. Whereas adult alcoholics, for example, may get cited for driving under the influence, adolescents may not suffer this consequence simply because they have not yet begun to drive.

Morrison and Smith consider drug-addicted adolescents to

be in need of "habilitation" rather than rehabilitation because they have yet to gain many adult skills.

Adolescent Denial

Most drug-addicted people, particularly adolescents, exhibit denial. It causes them to be unable to perceive themselves or others as they really are. Because of this self-deception, they begin to deceive others. Drug-addicted adolescents lie about their behaviors and feelings and hide them from those who might confront them about their drug use. They lie about their substance abuse, guard their supply of drugs, and appear in public in altered states of consciousness. They hide drugs for future use, are preoccupied with drugs, and continue to use drugs despite punishment, warnings, or advice. They have dysfunctional emotional involvements with others and feel anger, rage, and defensiveness about their drug use. They blame others for their problems, pity themselves, and attempt to control others. They intellectualize about their drug use, withdraw from people who care about them, and are chronically irresponsible.

Denial explains drug-addicted behavior that is otherwise unexplainable. For example, I had one patient, a 15-year-old boy, whose drug of choice was Scotchgard. He and his best friend had enjoyed inhaling it together on a regular basis. This ended when his friend suddenly had a cardiac arrest from the effect of the substance on his heart and subsequently died. My young patient stayed away from Scotchgard for two months, and then started using it again. He clearly understood that Scotchgard caused adverse consequences, but "not for him."

Effect on Development

Adolescents mature into young adults by completing a series of developmental stages. Completion of these stages can be delayed by up to two years or more in drug-abusing adolescents. This means that a chemically dependent 17-year-old may have the social and emotional maturity of a 15-year-old.

CONCLUSIONS

During adolescence, physical and psychological growth undergo significant development. A desire for peer acceptance is the hallmark of this stage of life. Risk-taking and sensation-seeking behaviors in this age group are normal, including experimenting with drugs.

Adolescents give a number of reasons for using drugs. The overwhelmingly predominant reason is that drugs make them feel good and they don't feel that drugs do them any harm.

A chemically dependent adolescent may have a delay of up to two years or more in his social and emotional maturity.

II

Drug Abuse Prevention

6

History

SOME EVIDENCE THAT DRUG ABUSE CAN BE PREVENTED

A significant body of evidence indicates that preventive measures do work. The most convincing evidence comes from our experience with cigarette smoking. Since 1964, when the Surgeon General's first report on the adverse health consequences of smoking was published, the smoking rate in the United States has declined from 42 percent of the adult population to about 26.5 percent. Quite clearly, the message has gotten across that you should not begin smoking and if you have, you should stop. This favorable response has occurred despite the fact that the tobacco industry annually spends billions of dollars in the United States alone on advertising and marketing tobacco products.

Educational efforts also appear to be having a favorable effect on the use of most illicit drugs as well, since we have seen that the number of people using them has declined over the last few years.

HISTORY OF PREVENTION EFFORTS

Preventing drug abuse is a complex and difficult activity, but one that is crucial to our society. Drug use and attempts to control it are apparently as old as civilization itself. For practical purposes, prevention programs have been directed at adolescents and pre-adolescent children.

The modern history of drug abuse prevention began in the 1960s in response to an increase in the number of American youth who were "turning on, tuning in, and dropping out." The earliest prevention programs relied on overblown and inaccurate risks of drug use; that is, scare tactics. They were ineffective because they impaired the credibility of those trying to prevent the drug use. Another early approach involved presenting factual medical, psychological, and social information in an attempt to encourage rational decisions about drug use.

In the early 1970s, programs began to focus on traits that appeared to distinguish drug users from nonusers. Studies suggested a relationship between drug use and variables such as low self-esteem, poor decision-making skills, and poor communication skills. Although no attempt was made to determine which came first, the traits or the drug use, it would seem likely that good skills in these areas would help increase children's ability to say no to alcohol and drugs. At about the same time, programs were developed that provided young people with a variety of alternatives to drug use, ranging from wilderness challenges to community service to drug-free rock concerts.

In the late 1970s, four new trends in prevention evolved: (1) the involvement of parents and communities in prevention efforts, (2) the false idea that some drugs, particularly marijuana, are not harmful when used responsibly, (3) recognition of the importance of peer pressure in drug use, and (4) the concept of approaching prevention at many different levels.

PREVENTION PROGRAMS

Schonberg, in a monograph published in 1988 by the American Academy of Pediatrics, discusses six types of prevention programs: (1) individual focus, (2) family focus, (3) peer group focus, (4) school focus, (5) community focus, and (6) larger social environment focus.

Individual Focus

Programs that focus on the individual believe that drug abuse arises out of six factors:

1. *Biological vulnerabilities.* This concept is based on the belief that some individuals are biologically more susceptible to becoming addicted than others, and that biological markers will eventually be found to identify these individuals. Once certain children have been determined to possess such a biological marker, they could then be targeted for specific prevention efforts. To date, such a biological marker has not been identified, although some studies appear promising. This concept is based on the biological model.

2. *Affective regulation.* This concept is based on the belief that individuals use drugs to self-medicate a variety of problems—depression, anxiety, boredom, loneliness—or that drug abuse is a symptom of a primary psychological disorder. Prevention efforts are directed at identifying individuals at risk and providing non-pharmacological treatment of their underlying problems. This concept is based on the psychological model.

3. *Knowledge deficits.* This concept is based on the belief that individuals use drugs because they do not know about the detrimental effects that drugs cause. Programs with this focus attempt to make young people more aware of the adverse medical, psychological, and social consequences of drug abuse. They assume that if young people were aware of these negative consequences they would make rational decisions not to use drugs.

4. *Life-skills deficits.* This concept is based on the belief that young people use drugs because they have specific life-skills

deficits, such as low self-esteem, poor decision-making skills, or poor communication skills. These programs attempt to correct these deficits.

5. *Invulnerability.* This concept is based on the belief that, although young people recognize the adverse consequences of drug use, they do not believe the risks apply to them, which is a form of denial. These programs focus on information that is of immediate interest to adolescents, such as the fact that smoking causes premature wrinkling of the face, or that drinking can lead to the loss of a driver's license.

6. *Sensation seeking.* This concept is based on the theory that young people have a natural tendency to seek new, exciting, and sometimes risky experiences. Programs with this focus seek to provide alternative highs.

Family Focus

Prevention programs focused on the family view drug abuse in terms of one or more of the following four factors:

1. *Family dynamics.* This concept considers the risk of drug abuse to be associated with factors such as parental permissiveness or inconsistency, loose family structure, harsh physical punishment, and poor family communication. Programs with this focus seek to improve parenting skills.

2. *Socialization deficit.* This concept considers the family to be the major socialization agent, and that many families fail to teach children such values as self-control, self-motivation, and self-discipline. Programs with this focus teach parents ways of structuring the home environment to increase the likelihood that children will develop these skills.

3. *Parental modeling.* This concept is based on the belief that children's early notions about drug use are learned by observing how parents behave with tobacco, alcohol, over-the-counter medications, prescription medications, and illicit drugs such as mari-

juana and cocaine. The goal of these programs is to change and improve parental behavior.

4. *Social control.* This concept is based on the assumption that parents have abdicated responsibilities for their children's drug use. Programs with this focus seek to get parents to reinstate social controls.

Peer Group Focus

Prevention programs that focus on peer groups consider drug abuse to be the result of the following three factors:

1. *Conformity.* This concept is based on the assumption that a desire to fit in with the crowd is a major concern of adolescents. It attempts to help young people resist peer conformity by programs such as the "just say no" campaign. Programs with this focus also attempt to teach young people that drug use is not the norm.

2. *Peer modeling.* This concept is based on the assumption that drug abuse is learned from peers. It attempts to counteract negative peer models by exposing young people to attractive, positive models who communicate an antidrug message.

3. *Peer influence.* This concept is based on the assumption that young people use drugs because peers pressure them to do so. This program teaches peer-pressure resistance skills.

School Focus

Programs that focus on schools address the following two factors:

1. *Deterrence.* Deterrence-based programs emphasize the importance of consistently enforcing school drug policies. They advocate a drug-free campus policy.

2. *Lack of knowledge.* This concept is based on the assumption that young people use drugs because they are unaware of the

medical, psychological, and social hazards of drug abuse. These programs attempt to mold attitudes and beliefs that do not support drug abuse.

Community Focus

Programs that focus on the community address one or more of the following factors:

1. *Availability.* Most community-based programs attempt to reduce the availability of drugs. Raising the drinking age to 21 years is an example of this principle.

2. *Social climate.* This concept is based on the assumption that drug abuse arises out of environmental factors. These programs include increased law-enforcement efforts, strong school prevention programs, concerned parents groups, and antidrug editorials in local newspapers.

3. *Social bonding.* This concept is based on the assumption that drug abuse results from some young people's failure to bond to social institutions and to their norms. Programs with this focus provide young people with opportunities to make positive contributions to the community and to develop positive social bonds as a result. They involve young people in community service programs such as historical restorations, programs for the elderly, and youth job services.

Larger Social Environment Focus

These programs are directed at the larger social environment in which young people live.

1. *Advertising.* For years, young people have been exposed, often during broadcasts of athletic events, to famous athletes advertising beers. Full pages of color in magazines advertise alcoholic beverages and cigarettes, associating them adventure,

sexual attractiveness, or sophistication. On average, children watch television about 20 hours a week. Television messages are clear: If you can't sleep, take a sleeping pill. If you have a headache, take a pain pill. A pill is available to solve every problem. The average child sees alcohol advertised on television 75,000 times before he or she is of legal drinking age.

Programs focused on advertising attempt to limit, reduce, or eliminate cigarette and alcohol advertising, to use advertisements that counteract cigarette and alcohol advertisements by lampooning popular advertisements, and to teach young people about advertising techniques to aid them in seeing through the messages in advertisements.

2. *Mass media*. These programs attempt to educate writers, producers, and directors about the drug messages their productions convey and to help these individuals present a more realistic picture of substance abuse.

CONCLUSIONS

Prevention measures have been shown to work. Over the years, a number of approaches have been used. These have focused on the individual, the family, the school, the community, and the larger social environment.

7

The Parent's Role

GENERAL SUGGESTIONS

To begin, let me say that nothing you do or, for that matter, don't do will guarantee that your children will never use drugs. There are, however, a number of steps you can take to reduce the likelihood that they will turn to drugs.

Learn about Drugs

Needless to say, it is not possible to take steps to prevent something if you don't know anything about what you are trying to prevent. Buying this book was a good start. Study it, save it, and refer back to it when the need arises.

Take other opportunities to learn about this subject. Make a special effort to watch television programs about drug abuse, attend local conferences on the subject when they are available, and read other material on the subject from time to time.

A significant part of this self-education is to learn what drug paraphernalia looks like and what it is used for. You should be able to recognize such items as roach clips, bongs, cocaine vials, and crack pipes. In addition, you should learn to recognize some of the commonly used drugs such as marijuana, LSD, amphetamines, and cocaine.

Once you have assembled your educational material, it should be reviewed by both you and your spouse so that the two of you can be consistent in your facts. If you are divorced, this is especially important because children of one-parent homes are at increased risk of developing alcohol and other drug problems. Recommended videos are given in Appendix C of this volume, and some recommended reading is indicated in the bibliography.

Teach Your Children about Drugs

Unfortunately, too many children receive their drug education outside of the home. Less than one-third of children learn about drugs from their parents. Nearly two-thirds learn about drugs from their friends. Some parents fail to teach their children about drugs out of neglect, while others do it because they wrongly fear that discussing drugs will condone their use. Another reason for parents' failing to teach their children about alcohol and other drugs is because they don't feel that they have enough expertise on the subject to do so.

As mentioned earlier, the primary reason adolescents give for using drugs is because drugs make them feel good and they do not believe that they will suffer adverse consequences from drug use. Parents who do not know specific facts about the various drugs tend to make statements such as, "Drugs will fry your brain." These kinds of statements are totally meaningless; all they do is impair credibility. If you want your children to really listen to you, you have to make statements that are true, meaningful, and specific, such as, "Cocaine can cause heart attacks in young people."

Here are some hints on teaching your children about drugs: First, never lecture, it only turns them off. Second, don't make the teaching sessions formal. Do the teaching during the dozens of natural opportunities that arise each week—when watching television together, when listening to the radio, when reading, in the car, or over the dinner table. These opportunities are known as *teachable moments*. Don't overwhelm them with too much informa-tion at any one time. If you have children of various ages, teach them individually and adapt your teaching level to their ages.

Third, use illustrations from books to show your children what the various drugs look like so they can knowledgeably decline should one be offered to them. Don't fail to acknowledge that drugs do give pleasurable effects. To do so would be dishon-est. Your children certainly would begin to wonder why so many people use them if they didn't; however, it is important for them to realize that the pleasure is short-lived and that prolonged drug use leads to extremely unpleasant results, destroying families and lives. In addition, one really does not know what he or she is getting when they buy illicit drugs. They are simply taking the dealer's word. It could just as well be sugar, or even worse, a poison. After all, how trustworthy can an individual be who is breaking the law to make money?

Fourth, when one uses drugs to get rid of his or her unhappi-ness, the relief is only temporary. When the drug wears off, the pain comes back, only worse since no actions have been taken to resolve the problem. With continued drug use, other problems develop, leading to more and more unhappiness. Children need to know this.

Fifth, make use of role models known to have used drugs. A number of professional athletes are recovering drug addicts who speak freely of their drug use and how it ruined, or nearly ruined, their lives. Some, such as the University of Maryland basketball star Lynn Bias, lost their lives from drug use. In addition, many rock musicians are now telling their stories about how drug abuse nearly destroyed them and how happy they are now to be drug-free.

Sixth, a good approach is to ask questions of your children, rather than always giving them fact after fact. For example, if you initiate a discussion about drugs and your child interrupts with, "Oh, I know all that stuff," counter them with, "Really? Tell me about it." The discussion can then be a two-way effort.

Seventh, teach your children about the possible legal consequences of drug use. Check with your local police and find out what the consequences are for being charged with possession of a controlled substance and for selling a controlled substance. The sentences vary from state to state. Being caught with a small amount of drug can get one anywhere from 2 to 10 years in prison in some states. Selling a drug in some states can result in penalties ranging from 15 years to life. This information can be pretty sobering to a child who sees very little wrong with drug use.

How early should you start teaching your children about drugs? Basically, you can't start too early. You certainly should start by the age of three or four. However, anytime up through preadolescence is better than never.

Recommended reading for children is given in Appendix B of this volume. Always be on the lookout for additional material to help you teach this subject to your children.

Forbid Drug Use

This should be a firm, fast rule in your family—no drugs of any kind. No tobacco products, no alcohol, and no marijuana or other illicit drugs. It is imperative that your children understand this.

1. *Be specific.* Explain the reasons for your rules about alcohol and other drugs. Discuss the consequences of breaking the rules: what the punishment will be, how it will be carried out, and what the punishment is supposed to achieve.

2. *Be consistent.* Make it clear to your child that the rules remain the same at all times: in your home, in a friend's home, or anywhere else the child happens to be.

3. *Be reasonable.* Don't add new consequences that have not been discussed before the rule was broken. When a rule is broken, react calmly and carry out the punishment that the child expects to receive for breaking the rule.

Teach Your Children about Advertising

Monitor what your children watch on television. Censorship is not necessary; however, you should take every opportunity to discuss the fallacy of the prodrug messages with your children. There are many reasons why the amount of time children spend watching television every day should be limited to less than two hours or so. Prodrug messages is but one.

Teach your children the common techniques used by advertisers to sell products. These include:

- *Bandwagon Approach.* This approach emphasizes that since everyone uses the product, so should you.
- *Snob Appeal.* This implies that only rich and famous people use this product.
- *Personal Testimony.* A respected celebrity tells you that he or she uses the product and it is wonderful.
- *Sex Appeal.* Beautiful people use this product, so if you want to be beautiful you should use it too.
- *Having Fun.* You will have lots of fun if you use this product. Your life will be better.
- *Comparison.* This product is better than other products. This claim may or may not be true.
- *Scare Tactics.* If you don't use this product, something bad will happen to you.

Examine Your Own Attitudes and Behaviors

Every family has expectations of behavior that are determined by principles and standards. These are known as *values*. Children who decide not to use alcohol or other drugs often do so because they have a strong conviction that the use of these substances, based on their value system, is wrong. Social, family, and religious values give young people reasons to say no and help them stick to their decision. You can make your family's values clear in various ways.

Recognize How Your Actions Affect the Development of Your Child's Values

Children copy their parents' behavior. How do you really feel about the use of tobacco, alcohol, marijuana, cocaine and other drugs? How do you manifest your feelings about these drugs? Do you have an ambivalent feeling about some, or all of them? Do you condone smoking and drinking, or even the use of marijuana? Remember, up until the beginning of adolescence, you have more influence on your child than anyone else in the world. What you think, what you say, and even more important, what you do has a profound effect on them.

Children can understand and accept that there are differences between what adults may do legally and what children may do. If you drink, keep the distinction sharp. Do not let your children be involved in your drinking by mixing you a cocktail, bringing you a beer, or having sips of your beer.

Look for Conflicts between Your Words and Your Actions

The old parental statement, "Do as I say, not as I do," is hypocritical. The fact is, your children are a lot more apt to do what you do than what you say.

Provide a positive role model. If you smoke, stop. Get help if you need it. If you drink, drink only in moderation, or better yet, quit. If you occasionally smoke marijuana or snort cocaine, you have little hope of raising drug-free children. The same goes for certain prescription medications. If you take Valium to help you deal with stress, Halcion to help you sleep, or Darvon for headaches or chronic pain, see your physician and ask him or her to arrange for nondrug, or at least nonaddicting drug, alternatives. If you are addicted to these drugs, you may need help getting off them.

You should clean out your medicine cabinet. Get rid of medications that have not been used in a long time or that are very infrequently used. A full medicine cabinet gives your child the message that it is okay to use drugs. Another reason for disposing of medications is that, for some children, your bathroom cabinet provides a convenient source of drugs.

Make Sure Your Child Understands Your Family Values

Parents sometimes assume that children absorb values even though they are never openly discussed. Discuss your family's values with your children. Do they know how you feel about honesty, integrity, self-reliance, and responsibility?

Examine Your Family Health

Does your family have healthy characteristics? Healthy characteristics include communicating and listening, respecting others, having a sense of trust, sharing responsibility, and admitting to and seeking help with problems. A healthy family is not perfect. Members go through illnesses, career crises, accidents, and losses that are part of normal living; however, they adjust to changes in a healthy manner. If your family health is not good, it is never too late to pursue this as a goal. Family counseling may be needed. Take whatever steps are necessary. Children growing up in healthy families are less likely to use drugs than those growing up in dysfunctional families; that is, families that do not possess healthy characteristics.

Examine Your Own Characteristics

Did you grow up in a dysfunctional family? Have you carried dysfunctional characteristics into your adult life? If you have, you may need counseling. If your family was dysfunctional because of alcoholism, you may need to join an Adult Children of Alcoholics group.

Promote Responsible Behavior

To develop responsible behavior, children must have something to be responsible for. At an early age, begin assigning age-related tasks. Young children can help you fold the clothes. Later, they can take out the garbage and help with the dishes. Older children can help prepare meals, mow the lawn, and do a variety of tasks around the house. Holding down a part-time job after school is a tremendous developer of responsible behavior.

Assign a time for adolescents to be home when they go out in the evening. When they start driving, expect responsible behavior behind the wheel. Realistic consequences should be established in advance when family rules are broken. Above all, be consistent. When you make a rule and it is broken, always follow through on seeing that your children suffer the consequences of their behavior. Parental inconsistency is deadly to the development of responsible behavior.

Promote Open Communication

This is an absolute must. Children should feel that they can discuss anything with you. You have to take the time to listen. Communication shows your children that you care. It requires work and involves a real commitment on your part. What you may find insignificant in your children's conversation may be of vital importance to them. Let your children know that they are more important to you than a football game on TV or a book. Talk about mundane things. How can you expect your children to talk to you about major topics in their lives if they have never talked to you about everyday occurrences? Ask about school, play, friends, or anything, and then listen. Remember: talking about her new doll or his new truck may be the most important thing in the world to your child.

Don't be afraid to admit that you don't have all the answers.

Let your child know that if you don't know an answer, you can work together to find one.

Here are some tips that will make talking with your child about alcohol and other drugs easier and more effective.

1. *Be a good listener.* Make sure your child feels comfortable bringing questions or problems to you. Listen carefully to what your child says. Don't interrupt. Don't prepare what you are going to say while your child is speaking. Reserve judgment until your child has finished speaking and is ready for your response.

Don't allow anger at what you hear to interfere with the discussion. If your child does not come to you with questions or problems, take the initiative. Ask about what is going on at school or in other activities.

2. *Give lots of praise.* Emphasize what your child is doing right instead of always focusing on things he does wrong. Parents that are quicker to praise than to criticize teach children to feel good about themselves and to develop self-confidence.

3. *Role-model good behavior.* Communication goes beyond just being verbal. Children learn by example as well. Make sure your own actions reflect the standard of honesty, integrity, and fair play that you expect of your child.

4. *Pay attention to nonverbal cues.* Be aware of your child's facial expression and body language. Does he seem nervous and uncomfortable or relaxed and comfortable? Reading these signs will let you know how your child is feeling.

During the conversation, acknowledge what your child is saying—move your body forward if you are sitting, touch a shoulder, or nod your head and make eye contact.

5. *Respond appropriately.* "I am very concerned about . . . " or "I understand that . . ." are better ways to respond to your child than beginning sentences with "You should . . ." or "When I was your age. . . ." If your child tells you something you would rather not hear, don't ignore the statement. Don't offer advice in response to every statement your child makes. Listen carefully to what is being said and try to understand the real feeling behind

the words. Be sure you understand what your child means. Respond when he is finished.

Promote Alternatives to Drug Use

Reasons adolescents give for using drugs include: recreation, as a socializer, for pleasure, and to relieve boredom. If you expect your child not to be tempted to use drugs, it is necessary for you to provide alternatives to drug use, something that is better than drugs.

Children should be exposed to as many activities as possible as early as possible. These may include reading, model airplane building, stamp collecting, painting, pets, gardening, video games, and sports. By all means, encourage the participation of your children's friends in these activities as well. A pool table or Ping-Pong table in the home can serve as a magnet to attract their friends to your home for recreation. Make your home a haven. Insist, however, that when other children are in your home, they abide by the household rules.

Support your child's involvement in school activities, sports, or music without always pressuring him to win or excel. Do things with your child. Children appreciate the time parents spend with them, even doing chores.

In addition, encourage your children, when they are old enough, to seek part-time employment. Besides promoting responsibility, being employed also serves in its own way as a recreation. By all means, don't let the television become your child's only form of recreation.

Help Develop Self-Esteem

The truth of the matter is, the greatest hazard to your children regarding drug use is peer pressure. A child's desire to be accepted by his peers, beginning in early adolescence, is probably the strongest motivating factor in his life. Unfortunately, using drugs is often a requirement for being accepted in some peer groups.

Children with positive self-images are better able to resist peer pressure. So how do you build self-esteem? You begin by never berating your children. They should be handled firmly, but with respect. Tasks which are too complex or difficult for successful completion should be avoided, and children should be praised for successful completion of tasks. The statement, "You can be proud of yourself," says a lot to a child. Praise them often, even for small accomplishments.

Avoid using labels and put downs such as, "You're not as smart as your brother" or "You never do anything right." If you tell your children that they are worthless, your words may come true. Avoid being angry with your children. Remember, it's the actions, not the person, that deserve the reprimand. Never punish them when you are angry. Don't expect your children to live up to the accomplishments of others. Let your children know that your love is unconditional, and that nothing they can do will make you stop loving them.

Teach Refusal Skills

The development of various peer pressure skills will prepare your child to say no to alcohol and other drugs.

Peer Pressure Skill 1. Teach your child to value individuality. Talk about people the child loves. Ask what makes them individuals. Ask your child what he likes about his own individuality. Add any good characteristics your child leaves out.

Peer Pressure Skill 2. Explore the meaning of friendship with your child. Ask your child to make a list of what a friend is and what a friend is not. Make a list of your own. When finished, make a game of seeing how many of the same characteristics you both have on your lists.

Peer Pressure Skill 3. Help your child avoid risky situations.

There are situations that encourage a child to drink or use other drugs. Make a rule that your child when he is young will not play at friends' homes when the parents are not at home, nor will he attend unchaperoned parties until he is older.

Peer Pressure Skill 4. Teach your child to use peer pressure. Some school systems and youth groups sponsor peer programs where children support each other's positive values. Inquire about such programs.

Peer Pressure Skill 5. Give your child the support needed to say no. While being polite, respectful, and agreeable are good traits in most situations, they do not prepare a child to be assertive. Tell your child that there are certain times one must insist on being taken seriously when he or she says no, especially when it comes to alcohol or other drugs.

Telling your children to "just say no" is inadequate. Having simply said "no," the pressure to use drugs does not normally stop. What does he or she do then? Other techniques your children can use are as follows: (1) be a broken record—say no repeatedly if pressure to use drugs continues, (2) state that "Drugs are not good for me. I am not interested," (3) change the subject, (4) suggest something else to do, and (5) leave if drugs are being used.

Role playing is an extremely effective tool. To role play, the parent pretends to be the drug-using friend and tries to get the child to agree to use a drug. The child practices responses to avoid doing so.

One of the reasons it is so difficult for a child to say no when a drug is offered is because it most often is done so by a friend or an older sibling. Less than 20 percent of children's primary drug sources are dealers.

Allow More Freedom in Decision Making

The primary tasks of parenting are helping children grow intellectually and emotionally, helping them become independent individuals, and finally, letting go. Parents should gradually loosen the reins of control as their children get older so that the children ultimately do not have to declare their independence in a self-destructive fashion.

Rebellion is one of the reasons adolescents give for using drugs. Don't force your children to rebel by being too strict and failing to gradually give them more and more freedom in making decisions. If your children are never given opportunities to make mistakes, how can they learn from them? You cannot live your children's lives for them. Sooner or later you are going to have to let go, voluntarily or involuntarily.

Monitor Friendships

Another way parents can deal with peer pressure is to have some input into who is providing it. It is important to get to know your children's friends. Up through the preteen years, this is relatively easy to do. They are all from the same neighborhood, and probably spend a lot of time in your home. Not only is it easy to get to know these friends, it is usually easy to get to know their parents as well.

When it comes to teenagers, however, the problem becomes much more difficult. Their circle of friends broadens because of two factors: (1) they graduate to larger secondary schools that combine children coming from several elementary schools, and (2) with the advent of a driver's license they venture farther from home, away from the neighborhood and the people you know.

When your adolescent meets new friends from other neighborhoods, arrange to get to know them. Suggest that your child invite them over to spend the night if they are of the same sex. Alternatively, invite them to dinner. When they come, talk to them. Get to know them. Appraise both their positive and negative characteristics. Weigh the balance of these in coming to a decision.

If you suspect that a child may indeed be a seriously negative influence on your youngster, check him out. If any of your other children know the child, discuss his or her reputation with them. If there is another couple you know with children in the same school, speak to them about your child's new friend. They may have some information.

If, after a thorough investigation, you come to the conclusion that the friend's behavior does indeed present a threat to your child's well-being, you have every right to forbid your child to see that person. Explain to your child the reasons behind the decision, the evidence you have that the friend is involved with alcohol or other drugs, and that this is not punishment. Once you have made the decision, stick to it. Explain to your child that if a friend insists that you drink or use drugs, that person is not a very good friend. A true friend would respect your decision.

Set Limits and Consequences

Children want structure in their lives. They behave more responsibly when parents set limits. They need to know where what they can do ends and what they can't do begins. Set clear and appropriate limits and enforce them. The limits should be written and all parties concerned should discuss them to be sure that everyone is in agreement as to what they mean. They should then be posted where you and your children can easily see them.

Consequences for going beyond the limits should also be discussed and their meaning agreed on. They too should be posted. Consequences should be related to the incident, be reasonable, timely, and not too elaborate, escalate in force with repeated infractions, applied consistently, and enforced calmly, respectfully, and without anger. Consequences should be looked at as acts of love. Seeking revenge for having been disobeyed, making threats, and shaming should be avoided. These behaviors serve no positive purpose.

Be Conscious of Mood States

Adolescents also state that they use drugs in response to stress, anxiety, and depression. Adolescence is a stressful state, and anxiety is common. Self-medicating this mood state may seem appropriate, especially if the adolescent has grown up in a home in which the philosophy has been to take a pill for every unpleasant feeling.

Depression, too, can lead to drug use, although it is more often the result of it. Look for psychosomatic illnesses such as headaches or stomachaches, as well as weight gain or loss, changes in mood or behavior, and self-destructive behavior. The depression may also be masked as anger.

Barun and Bashe identify seven common causes of adolescent depression, listed in order of severity: (1) a family's decision to move, (2) poor communication with parents, (3) family's money problems, (4) beginning and end of the school year, (5) mother's pregnancy, (6) parental separation or divorce, and (7) death of a parent. Be especially aware of your children's mood states in these situations. Should stress, anxiety, or depression reach abnormal states, do not hesitate to consult a psychologist or psychiatrist.

Develop Parental Agreement

It is absolutely essential that both parents agree on what steps will be taken to prevent drug abuse. Drug abuse is more common in single-parent families. Because relations are often strained between the ex-partners, they often fail to concur on behavior standards for their children. No matter how awkward, however, both parents should cooperate. It is in the child's best interest that the absent parent consistently support the at-home parent's anti-drug efforts.

Get Involved

By all means, get involved in neighborhood parent groups, school activities, and community programs that attempt to prevent drug abuse. Share drug education materials, work together to coordinate curfews, pressure schools to institute drug policies and drug prevention programs, and pressure establishments that sell cigarettes and alcoholic beverages to minors to stop doing so.

AGE-SPECIFIC PREVENTION EFFORTS

The preceding section of this chapter outlined some general suggestions about how to reduce the likelihood that your child will use alcohol or other drugs. The messages can be more effective if you take into account the knowledge your children already have and their readiness to learn new information at different ages.

Ages Three through Four

The knowledge and attitudes learned early can have an important effect on the decisions children make later. Although children in this age group cannot learn complex facts about alcohol and other drugs, they can begin to learn the decision-making and problem-solving skills that will be needed to refuse drugs. Remember that children in this age group are not able to listen quietly for very long. They are more interested in doing things for themselves. Make use of this characteristic.

Suggested Activities

Set aside regular times when you can give your child your full attention. Activities such as playing together, reading a book, and taking a walk help to build strong bonds of trust and affection that will help reduce the influence of peer pressure in the adolescent years.

Explain how medicines can be harmful if used inappropriately. Teach your child not to take anything from a medicine bottle unless you give it to him yourself or specify someone else who can give it.

Explain why children should put only good things into their bodies. Explain how good foods will make their bodies healthy. A focus on healthy bodies will help them avoid putting harmful things like drugs into their bodies when they are older.

Take advantage of opportunities to use play as a way of helping your child learn to handle frustrating situations and solve simple problems. Turning a bad situation into a success reinforces a child's self-confidence. This will help him say no to peer pressure later.

Help your child learn decision-making skills. For example, give him a choice of two or three shirts and let him decide which to wear. Let your child know that you think he is able to make good decisions.

Ages Five through Nine

Five- to nine-year-olds still learn through experience and don't have a good understanding of things that will happen in the future. Children in this age group need rules to guide their behavior and information to make good decisions.

Discussions about alcohol and other drugs must be in the here and now and related to events the child knows about. Children in this age range still do not possess good abstraction skills.

Helping your child know whom to trust is important. They need to learn that just because someone tells them to do something, it is not always right to do it.

By age nine, your child should understand:

- what an illicit drug is, why it is illegal, what it looks like, and what harm it can do
- what alcohol and nicotine are and how they can be harmful
- how poisons, medicines, and illicit drugs differ

- how medicines can help when used appropriately and how they can be harmful when misused
- why it is important to avoid ingesting unknown substances
- what school and home rules are about alcohol, nicotine, and other drug use
- why using alcohol and nicotine is illegal for children

Suggested Activities

1. Explain the need for rules by talking about how traffic safety rules help us.

2. Emphasize the importance of good health. You can use this discussion to stress how using drugs, smoking, or drinking to excess can do harmful things to the body.

3. Discuss how TV advertisements try to persuade people to buy products and how they should use their own judgment about whether or not the items advertised are good for them or if they are even things they want. This will help them understand how to respond to beer commercials and cigarette advertisements when they are older.

4. Discuss illnesses with which your child is familiar (earaches, colds, sore throats) and for which prescription medication may be necessary. Discussing such illnesses can help your child understand the difference between medicines and illicit drugs.

5. Practice ways to say no with your child. Give him or her some responses to use in various situations. Role playing can be helpful.

Ages 10 through 12

Children aged 10 to 12 years love to learn facts and how things work. Studies have shown that the earlier children begin to use drugs, the more likely they are to have serious problems in the future. It is not uncommon for 6th graders to be offered alcohol and other drugs. Increased efforts focusing on drug-use prevention are warranted.

Appropriate new information should include:

- ways to identify specific drugs, including alcohol, tobacco, marijuana, inhalants, and cocaine in their various forms
- the long- and short-term consequences of drug use
- the effects of drugs on different parts of the body and the reasons why drugs are especially dangerous for growing bodies
- the consequences of alcohol and other drug use to families, society, and the user

Suggested Activities

1. Create special times when you are available to talk with your child, such as a walk, a visit to the ice cream parlor, or after a movie. This will help you to continue to build your relationship so that some of the inevitable peer pressure, when it occurs, can be somewhat defused.

2. Encourage your child to participate in activities like sports, scouting, or religious-sponsored youth activities. Such activities allow him to make new friends and develop nondrug-using pastimes.

3. Teach your child how the use of alcohol and cigarettes is promoted to be glamorous, when in fact it is not.

4. Continue to practice ways of saying no with your child. Emphasize ways to refuse alcohol and other drugs. Again, role playing can be a useful tool.

5. Encourage your child to join a local antidrug club if one is available.

6. Ask your child to scan the newspaper and circle articles which have to do with alcohol or other drug use. Articles about drug-related murders, alcohol-related automobile accidents, or drug-related arrests appear regularly.

7. Make friends with the parents of your children's friends so that you can reinforce one another's antidrug efforts.

8. Join with other parents in providing supervised activities for young people to limit free time. Too much free time often leads to experimenting with alcohol or other drugs.

Ages 13 through 15

Fitting in with friends is of major importance to children in their early teens. The decision-making and problem-solving skills your child learned earlier can be very important.

Children in this age group are beginning to learn to deal with abstractions and the future. They understand that their actions have consequences and know how their behavior affects others. Strong emotional support and good adult role modeling are very important.

Telling 13-year-olds that they will get lung cancer or heart disease in 30 to 40 years if they smoke is fruitless. Messages have to be about the here and now. Emphasize the bad breath, stained teeth, and early facial wrinkling that smoking causes.

In this age range, reinforce the no-alcohol/no-drug use rules. Be sure your child understands clearly that alcohol, cigarettes, and other drugs are illegal and that breaking the law is unacceptable behavior.

By age 15, your child should know:

- the characteristics of specific drugs
- the effects of drugs on the circulatory, respiratory, nervous, and reproductive systems
- the stages of chemical dependence (use, abuse, dependence) and their unpredictability from person to person
- the ways drug use affects activities requiring coordination, such as driving a car or participating in sports
- the role of family history in the risk of becoming addicted to alcohol and other drugs

Suggested Activities

1. Get to know your child's friends and their parents. Share your expectations about behavior. Work together to develop a set of rules about curfews, unchaperoned parties, and other social activities. Stick together.

2. Monitor your child's whereabouts. If your child is going to a movie, be sure you know what movie is playing, at which theater, and who he is going with. Last-minute changes in plans, such as going to a different movie, should not be permitted unless the child checks with you or another designated adult.

3. Continue to practice ways to say no with your child. Teach him to recognize problem situations such as being in a house where no adults are present and where drinking beer is taking place, and how to handle them.

4. Your child's fears about such things as emerging sexuality and appearing different from friends deserve your concern and attention. Spend time with your child to discuss feelings about things that are felt to be important to him.

5. Periodically review and update, with your child's participation, your house rules and your child's responsibilities regarding chores, time watching TV, and curfews.

6. Teach your child that true friends do not ask each other to do things that are wrong and which might risk harm to themselves, their friends, or their families.

7. Plan supervised parties, such as having your child invite friends to share a pizza and watch TV.

Ages 16 through 18

High school students are future-oriented and can engage in abstract thinking. They have increasingly realistic understanding of adults and become more interested in the welfare of others. Belonging to the group continues to motivate much of their behavior.

By the end of high school, your child should understand:

- both the immediate and long-term physical effects of specific drugs
- the possible fatal outcome of combining drugs
- the relationship of drug use to diseases and disabilities
- the effect of alcohol and other drugs on the fetus during pregnancy
- the relationship between drug use and AIDS
- the possible consequences of operating equipment, including automobiles, while under the influence of alcohol and other drugs
- the impact of alcohol and other drugs on society

Suggested Activities

1. Focus on the potential long-term effects of alcohol and other drugs, such as ruining a chance of getting into college, being hired for certain jobs, or getting into the military.

2. Impress on your child the importance of serving as a good role model for a younger brother or sister.

3. Keep your child involved in family activities such as dinner, vacations, and family routines.

4. Plan strategies to limit your child's unsupervised time at home. The time between three o'clock and six o'clock p.m. is particularly dangerous for drug experimentation.

5. Encourage your child to work on behalf of a drug prevention program if one is available.

6. The busier your child is the less likely he is to get involved with alcohol and other drugs. Talk with him about joining organizations, such as a sports club or an arts and crafts center, or volunteering to work for a church group or community organization.

7. Plan alcohol- and drug-free activities with other families

during school vacations, which can be high-risk times for teenagers.

8. Make an effort to be informed about new drugs that are popular and learn about their effects and dangers.

9. Help plan community-sponsored drug-free activities, such as dances and other recreational activities.

OTHER PREVENTION EFFORTS

Strong policies that spell out rules governing the use, possession, and sale of alcohol and other drugs should be a key part of school-based prevention programs. Learn what your child's school policies are and actively support them. If your child's school has no policy, work with teachers, administrators, and community members to develop one. Good school policies typically specify what constitutes an alcohol or other drug offense, spell out the consequences for violating the policy, and describe procedures for handling violations.

Visit your child's school and learn how drug education is being taught. Is it taught only in the health class, or is it incorporated into all subject areas? Do children in every grade receive drug education or is it limited to a few grades?

If your child's school has a drug-abuse prevention program, ask to see the materials that are being used. Does the school have referral sources for students who need help?

Community–Parent Cooperation

Support community efforts to give young people healthy alternatives. Alcohol- and drug-free proms and other school-based celebrations are growing in popularity. Local businesses can offer support through athletic events and part-time jobs.

CONCLUSIONS

You, as a parent, can do a number of things to increase the likelihood that your children will remain drug-free. These things are more effective when they take into account the age of the child.

You can also get involved in your child's school drug-abuse prevention program. If the school does not have such a program, you can take steps to get one started. You can also work with business leaders in a drug-abuse prevention effort.

8

The Teacher/Counselor's Role

GENERAL SUGGESTIONS

As a teacher or a counselor, you can engage in many of the same types of prevention efforts described for parents in the previous chapter. You can:

- learn about drugs
- be cognizant of teaching opportunities at school
- support your school's no-drug policy if it has a formal one
- examine your own attitudes about the use of alcohol and other drugs
- promote responsible behavior
- promote alternatives to drug use
- help develop self-esteem
- allow more freedom in decision-making
- be conscious of mood states
- get involved

If your school has a formal drug policy, support it. If not, push for the establishment of one. A school drug policy should state unequivocally that no drug use, possession, or sale is tolerated on school grounds at any time, including after class and on weekends. Schools should have a procedure for handling violations, and should follow it.

If your school has a drug-abuse prevention program, support it. If it does not have one, work with school officials and parents to get one started.

Antidrug education should start in kindergarten and continue through the 12th grade. In addition to the usual classroom activities such as lectures, films, readings, individual projects, and group work, teachers can invite local physicians, alcohol and drug counselors, recovering addicts, and police to their classrooms. They can also organize field trips to drug-rehabilitation facilities and police stations.

Distribute drug education literature to parents. The school should hire a counselor knowledgeable in substance abuse or train a member of the staff for the job. Older student volunteers can teach younger children.

The implementation of direct teaching methods such as lectures, films, readings, individual projects, and field trips along with the use of indirect teaching methods such as role playing and other group activities makes for the best drug-abuse prevention curriculum strategy. You already possess skills to implement the direct teaching activities. More difficult and more challenging is the teaching of attitudes and behavioral skills through indirect methods. When the primary goal of a curriculum is the development of attitudes and behavioral skills, the teacher becomes more of a teacher of people than a teacher of a subject. Facilitation of learning replaces the imparting of information. To do this effectively, it is absolutely necessary to build a climate of trust in which students feel free to share experiences and feelings without fear of being rebuffed.

Parents, teachers, and counselors should meet periodically to evaluate the effectiveness of the program.

SPECIFIC ATTITUDES AND SKILLS

General Recommendations

There are attitudes and skills you can cultivate to successfully conduct a drug-abuse prevention program:

- recognize learning experiences in the community which would make valuable contributions to the program
- admit when you do not know the answer
- refer counseling problems beyond your competence to appropriate resources
- recognize that your own personal alternatives to drug use, such as religion, might not be acceptable to everyone
- convey personal attitudes about alcohol and other drugs in a nonauthoritarian, nonlecturing manner
- accept reactions from students who do not agree with your position
- express interest in current issues, trends, and use patterns regarding drugs
- design and conduct classroom activities, such as role playing and group discussion, that give students the opportunities to develop and examine various ways of handling drug use issues
- recognize that family behavior and cultural mores may differ, and that what is right for one student is not right for all
- provide emotional support to students who disclose personal drug-abuse problems

Communication Skills

To influence children's attitudes about the abuse of alcohol and other drugs, it is first necessary to communicate with them effectively.

General Suggestions

The following are some general suggestions that have been proven helpful.

- Don't guess at what a child is feeling. Use good listening skills to determine the problem.
- Don't depend on nonverbal communication alone to get children to change their behavior. Also tell them what you want.
- Be aware of your nonverbal messages when having a discussion with a child
- Don't fold your arms in front of you when talking with a child. This indicates a closed mind
- Do express your feelings and wants to children, negative or positive
- Allow children in your class to ask you questions about yourself, but reserve the right to keep some things private. Honor their right to privacy. This gives them the feeling that you like them.
- Make a list of positive words you can use to compliment or give praise, and use these words often. Some examples are:

That's great!	Good job!
I am very proud of the way you worked today.	You are right!
	That is an excellent observation.
You can be proud of yourself for doing such a good job.	Very good!
	Excellent work!
	Good point!

- Don't preach. It is ineffective. Preaching involves using words like should, always, never, and ought. It gives a child the feeling that he is one of a number rather than an individual.
- Don't command. Ordering children to do things and threatening punishment eventually leads to sneaky, rebellious behavior.

- Avoid giving advice. The advice-giver tells children what to do in a kinder way than commanding; however, it discourages independent learning and creative thinking.
- Develop a list of feelings. This can be helpful as you encourage students to explore their feelings. Examples are

Happy	Sad	Angry	Scared	Confused
Joyful	Depressed	Furious	Terrified	Bewildered
Thrilled	Gloomy	Enraged	Nervous	Disorganized
Pleased	Dejected	Irate	Anxious	Foggy
Delighted	Heartbroken	Teed-off	Petrified	Mixed-up
Glad	Blue	Mad	Afraid	Puzzled

Listening Skills

There are five listening skills, known as *facilitation*, that can improve communication with children:

1. Rephrase the child's comments to show you understand. This is sometimes called *reflective listening*. It serves three purposes: (1) it assures the child that you hear what he is saying, (2) it allows the child to rehear what he has said, and (3) it assures that you correctly understand the child's comments.

2. Watch the child's face and body language. A child may tell you that he does not feel sad, but a quivering chin can tell you otherwise. When words and body language say two different things, always believe the body language.

3. Give nonverbal support and encouragement. This may consist of a gentle touch, a pat on the shoulder, making eye contact, or nodding your head.

4. Use the appropriate tone of voice for the answer you give. Your voice tone communicates as clearly as your words. Be sure your tone does not come across as disinterested, irritated, sarcastic, or all-knowing.

5. Use encouraging words or phrases to show your interest and keep the conversation going. Spoken at appropriate times,

such as during pauses in the conversation, these words or phrases can communicate to the child that you are interested in what is being said.

Self-Esteem Building Skills

Development of a positive self-image will allow children to more effectively deal with peers who pressure them to use alcohol or other drugs. Here are five self-esteem building skills you can use:

1. Give lots of praise, for effort as well as accomplishment. Look for achievement even in small tasks, and praise the child often. It is important to communicate the concept that doing one's best is more important than winning.

2. Help the child set realistic goals. If expectations are too high, the resulting failure can be detrimental to self-esteem.

3. Criticize the action, not the child. When the child does an act that is dangerous, of poor judgment, or against the rules, be sure the action gets the criticism. Incorrect response—"You shouldn't have jumped off that wall. Don't you have any sense?" Correct response—"Jumping off that wall was dangerous. You could have been hurt. Please don't do it again."

4. Give the child real responsibility. Children who have regular responsibilities learn to see themselves as part of a team. Completing the duties gives them a sense of accomplishment.

5. Show children you care about them. An occasional hug helps a child feel good about himself. Children are never too old to be told that they are valued.

Coping Skills

Everyone, no matter how old he is, cares about what other people think, and wants to fit in. As children approach adolescence, peer pressure becomes an ever-increasing influence on the way they feel, act, dress, and behave. The pressure to go along with the crowd can be either good—joining a club, playing sports, making good grades—or bad—smoking cigarettes, skipping school, or shoplifting. It takes courage for a child to stand up for what he believes, especially when it means going against what a friend wants him to do. Children should be taught that real friends want them to be themselves.

Most children are introduced to drugs by their peers, friends, brothers, sisters, and acquaintances. The pressure exerted to use drugs may be direct or indirect. Direct pressure usually consists of one or more peers trying to get a child to try a drug. Indirect pressure is more subtle. For example, a child may be at a party where a joint is being passed around, and even though no one asks him to smoke, he may feel pressured to join in, to be one of the crowd.

Assertive Behavior

To say no, a child must learn to be assertive. Assertive behavior is:

• behavior which allows someone to act in his own best interest, to stand up for himself without undue anxiety, and to exercise his rights without denying the rights of others.
• not aggressive behavior. It does not violate the rights of others. For example, letting someone know you are angry at the time the feeling occurs is assertive. Degrading the other person because you feel angry is aggressive.
• not allowing yourself to be taken advantage of because of not saying no. Children fail to be assertive because the other person might not like them anymore, get mad, do something to get revenge, feel hurt or guilty, or cry.

Assertive behavior allows you to reduce your need for someone else's approval, reduces social anxiety, develops communication which can result in closer friendships and more intimate relations, and increases self-respect.

Usually there are three basic components in the content of assertive behavior: (1) recognition of the other person's feelings or rights, (2) expression of one's own feelings and rights, and (3) description of the desired action.

Assertive behavior consists of the content of a response (what is said) as well as how it is said (*nonverbal behavior*). Nonverbal behavior includes eye contact, body posture, and vocal tone.

Verbal Assertive Responses

There are nine types of verbal assertive responses:

1. *Assertive talk*: used to prevent others from taking advantage of you. Examples are "I was here first," "I'd like more coffee please," "Please turn down your radio," and "Excuse me, I have another appointment."

2. *Feeling talk*: these responses express your likes and dislikes. Examples are "What a beautiful blouse," "I'm tired," and "I much prefer you in another type of outfit."

3. *Greeting talk*: don't avoid people because of shyness or because of not knowing what to say. Be outgoing and friendly with people you would like to know. Examples are "Hi, how are you?," "Hello, I haven't seen you in months," and "Taking any good courses?"

4. *Disagreeing passively and actively*: if you disagree with someone, don't feign agreement by smiling, nodding, or paying close attention. Change the topic, look away, disagree actively and emotionally.

5. *Asking why*: when asked to do something by a person in authority that does not sound reasonable, ask why you should do it, and request an explanation.

6. *Talking about oneself*: if you have done something worthwhile or interesting, you should let others know about it. Don't

monopolize the conversation, but don't be afraid to insist on your turn to talk either.

7. *Agreeing with compliments*: don't deprecate yourself when complimented by another. Reward others rather than punishing them for giving you a compliment. For instance, you could say, "That's an awfully nice thing to say. I appreciate it."

8. *Looking people in the eye*: when arguing, expressing an opinion, or greeting a person, look the person directly in the eye.

9. *Saying no*: when a request is unreasonable and you feel your rights are being denied, or when you feel you are being taken for granted, you should say "no!" Offer other suggestions. Don't be defensive.

Nonverbal Assertive Responses

Nonverbal assertive responses include eye contact and facial expression, body posture and movement, and vocal tone and quality.

• *Eye contact and facial expression*: the person you are talking to is more likely to respond if you look him right in the eye. Appropriate expression lends credibility to your assertions.

• *Body posture and movement*: the more relaxed you are, the more comfortable you will feel being assertive. Turning away from the other person or lowering your head conveys a mixed message. Appropriate gestures lend credibility to an assertion.

• *Vocal tone and quality*: smooth rhythmic statements convey more confidence than a low, faltering voice.

Assertiveness, Aggressiveness, and Passive Behavior

These are three distinctly different behaviors.

1. *Assertiveness*. This is giving the message of what you think or feel. The goal is communication, not domination. Attempt to get what you want without violating the rights of others.

Nonverbal factors include posture (holding your head up and keeping your back straight), gestures (natural hand movements), voice tone (firm and audible), eye contact (short breaks), and facial expression (pleasant, smiling from time to time, serious when appropriate).

Assertiveness leads to positive responses such as problem resolution, improved relationships, reduction of anxiety and anger, and improved self-esteem.

2. *Aggressiveness.* This involves overpowering, humiliating, degrading, and threatening another. It conveys the message, "What I want is all that counts. You don't matter." The goal is to get what you want no matter who is hurt.

Nonverbal factors include posture (nose in the air, leaning forward into another person's face), gestures (pounding fist, pointing or shaking finger), voice tone (shouting), eye contact (staring), and facial expressions (threatening, scornful).

Negative consequences include losing friends, making enemies, causing others to seek revenge, and getting into fights.

3. *Passive behavior.* This involves letting others take advantage of you by not expressing your feelings, thoughts, and beliefs. People with passive behavior are often described as shy, meek, or timid. The message is, "I don't count. You can take advantage of me."

Nonverbal factors include posture (slouching, head hanging), gestures (wringing hands, twisting hair, biting pen), voice tone (soft), eye contact (avoiding eye contact), and facial expressions (constant smile, biting lip).

Negative consequences include loss of self-respect, being taken advantage of, and psychosomatic problems (headaches, ulcers).

Decision-Making Skills

Decision making is a process in which one chooses from among two or more possible choices. Personal decision making allows one to reason through life situations, to solve problems, and to modify behaviors. A decision is judged as effective or ineffective by whether it produces satisfying or nonsatisfying consequences. Particularly when one has important decisions to make, personal values are a major factor in what decisions are finally made.

Decision making is a logical process that can be followed in thinking the problem through and making the wisest decision.

Steps in the Decision-Making Process

The process for personal decision making consists of five steps:

1. *Defining the problem.* In this step, decide specifically what the problem is. Questions asked include: What is the problem? Whose problem is it? What information do I need to make a decision or solve the problem?

2. *Looking at influences.* In this stage, you examine the influences and pressures operating on your decision and their importance. For example, who or what is influencing my decision? You should also gather information about the problem in the form of facts and other people's opinions. Examine your own emotions about the problem and consider how they will affect the decision.

3. *Identifying alternatives.* Review a variety of choices along with the facts needed to weigh the different alternatives. Ask yourself: What choices do I have? Consider the influences operating on each possibility.

4. *Looking at risks and results.* Consider the various alternatives in light of what is likely to happen and what the benefits and risks are for each. Questions asked should include: What will happen as the result of each possible choice? What are the possible benefits? What are the possible costs or negative outcomes?

5. *Deciding, acting, and evaluating.* In this final step, one looks at the results of past decisions to guide future action. To help evaluate a decision, seven questions are asked: (1) What decision did I make in the past, and what action, thought, or feeling

resulted from that decision? (2) How satisfied am I with the result? (3) What cost did I expect from the decision? (4) What did I have to give up? (5) What positive outcome did I expect to get from the decision? (6) What were the actual costs and positive outcomes? (7) What would I do differently next time, and would I make that same decision now if I could turn back the clock?

SMALL GROUP WORK

Two small group activities of value in a drug-abuse prevention curriculum are small group discussions and role playing.

Small Group Discussions

The small group discussion technique is familiar to most teachers. It can be a useful mechanism for developing a project, an oral report, a bulletin board, a written paper, or a demonstration related to drugs, drug abuse, or drug abuse prevention.

Groups made up of four to six members encourage more individual participation. They work best when task oriented. Groups should be arranged so that there is a mix of sexes, talkers, and quiet students.

Teachers, sometimes with class input, should provide a list of acceptable group behaviors. Items on the list might include respecting one another's thoughts and ideas, allowing only one person to talk at a time, and no put-downs of another's ideas. One student may be appointed to keep the group focused on the task at hand.

The teacher can move from group to group, act as a resource person, and facilitate and encourage group work. The teacher should interrupt only when absolutely necessary.

The steps to follow in developing the small group investigation are:

1. The students encounter a problem situation. This can be planned by the teacher or unplanned.
2. The students explore their reactions to the situation.
3. The students and the teacher formulate the task and organize it for study.
4. The teacher provides time for group study and work. Group work proceeds.
5. The teacher and students analyze progress and processes and adjust and correct as necessary.
6. Student groups report on completed projects.

Role Playing

There are nine basic steps to be considered when putting together a role-playing situation:

1. *Warm up the group.* This consists of identifying the problem, making the problem explicit, interpreting the problem story, and exploring the issues. You should be sure to explain role playing if students have not done it before.

2. *Select participants.* Role selection is a critical decision-making activity. You may ask for volunteers, select students for the roles by chance, or choose certain students for certain roles. Don't exclude shy students. They may emerge as good role players by coming out of their shells.

3. *Set the stage.* Prepare the role players. Set up the situation and explain how each fits into the scenario.

4. *Prepare the observers.* The observers should be given specific instructions on what to look for.

5. *Enact the role play.* During the role play, you should make mental notes for use in the analysis part of the activity.

6. *Discuss and evaluate.* Review the role play (events, positions taken, realism). Discuss the major focus. Have the observers give their reports. Discuss the possibilities and the variables that might

change if a part of the role play were changed. Discuss the consequences.

7. *Reenactment.* Change the role players and remind the observers of their tasks. Repeat the role-playing activity. Have the observers note similarities and differences.

8. *Discuss and evaluate again.* See Step 6.

9. *Share experiences and generalize.* Relate the problem situation to real experiences and current problems. Explore general principles of behavior.

In role playing, you are responsible for initiating the steps and guiding students through the activities in each step. The content of the discussions and enactments is determined largely by the students.

Other teacher behaviors connected with role playing include (1) accepting all student responses in a nonevaluative manner, (2) helping students' awareness of their views and feelings by reflecting, summarizing, and paraphrasing their responses, (3) helping students explore various sides of the problem situation and compare alternative views, and (4) emphasizing that there are alternate ways to resolve any problem.

In a role-playing situation, one can choose a role that is a reversal of one's true-life situation. For instance, the child can be the parent. The student can be the teacher. The boy can be the girl. Since the situation is merely a simulated one, the role player can experience the role without fear of penalty for failure. Despite its low-risk potential, the opportunities for learning and growth are great.

GRADE-SPECIFIC CURRICULUM

A grade-specific drug-abuse prevention curriculum begins in kindergarten with simple factual information and concepts and progressively becomes more complex through the 12th grade. It is composed of learning components, goals, objectives, vocabulary terms, activities, and evaluations.

The learning components include information, self-esteem skills, coping skills, and decision-making skills. The goals are broad statements of what is to be accomplished. The objectives are specific measurable accomplishments designed to achieve the goals. A goal may have one or more objectives. Each objective is accompanied by specific vocabulary terms and activities.

Examples of Curriculum Components

Information

The purpose of this component is to transmit information about drugs, drug abuse, and the effects of drugs on individuals, families, and society. Consider the following example from the kindergarten portion of a curriculum:

GOAL: The student will demonstrate knowledge of the basic body parts.

OBJECTIVES: The student will

- name the major parts of the body
- illustrate the functions of each body part
- describe the healthy care of the body parts

VOCABULARY: Terms for the first objective above, for example, include

- Heart
- Stomach
- Brain
- Intestines
- Lungs
- Liver

ACTIVITIES: Activities associated with the first objective above include:

- Discuss that we can see some of our body parts (arms, eyes, hands, feet) but that some of our body parts cannot be seen because they are beneath the skin (heart, lungs, stomach).

- Have the students stand and play "Simon Says," naming visible body parts.
- Distribute a handout—a diagram of body and major parts—and have students color specific body parts:

Heart: red
Brain: blue
Lungs: yellow
Stomach: green
Intestines: orange
Liver: gray

Self-Esteem Skills

The purpose of this component is to help students develop a positive self-concept to better resist pressure to use alcohol or other drugs. Consider the following example from the Grade 3 portion of a curriculum.

GOAL: The student will demonstrate an appreciation for individual differences.

OBJECTIVES: The student will

- discuss ways in which individuals differ
- discuss benefits derived from individual differences
- illustrate how individual differences are shown through communication

VOCABULARY: Terms for the first objective above, for example, include

- individual differences
- unique

ACTIVITIES: Activities associated with the first objective above include:

- Introduce the term "individual differences." Ask the class for a definition. List all of the responses. Explain that "individual differences" refers to all of the ways in which each person is different from all other people and is, therefore, unique. Go back over the list of definitions and decide as a class if the originally generated list of responses still applies.
- List examples of ways in which individuals may differ; for example, height, likes, dislikes, abilities, living situation, musical ability, family size and make-up, strengths, and sound of voice.
- Discuss possible benefits from the fact that we all possess individual differences.
- Distribute a handout, "Self-Notes." This is an exercise in which students list some things themselves. The completed list can be sung to the tune of *Do, Re, Me, Fa, So, La, Ti, Do. DO* something, I can do well; *RE*member, a memorable moment; *ME*aningful, something very meaningful to me; *FA*vorite, my favorite thing; *SO*lo, something I do for myself; *LA*ughter, something that makes me laugh; *TI*me, the best time of my day; *DO*uble, something I do with someone else. Point out that some students are familiar with the musical scale while others may not be.

Coping Skills

The purpose of this component is to develop coping skills that will allow students to deal with various factors that tend to lead to use of alcohol or other drugs. Consider the following example from the Grade 5 portion of a curriculum.

GOAL: The student will demonstrate the ability to resolve peer conflict.

OBJECTIVES: The student will

- identify feelings and behaviors associated with peer pressure
- generate alternatives for resisting peer pressure
- explore situations in which peer conflict manifests itself

VOCABULARY: Terms for the first objective above, for example, include

- passive   • assertive
- aggressive   • pressure

ACTIVITIES: Activities associated with the first objective above include:

- Write on the board "passive, aggressive, assertive." Tell students that these words are used to describe three types of behaviors that people may exhibit when responding to pressure imposed by others.
- Behavior (body posture, eye contact, voice tone) plus content (what you actually say) are both equally important when responding to peer pressure. Discuss each type of response and model the behaviors and verbalizations for each.
- Distribute a handout, "How to Say No and Mean It." This is a list of the techniques to follow when confronted with pressure to use alcohol or another drug (discussed in the previous chapter). Discuss when saying no assertively would be important; for example, when someone is pressuring you to do something you do not want to do, such as use a drug. Discuss each of the techniques for saying no. Discuss possible responses.

- Distribute a handout "Role-Plays." This exercise consists of five situations in which a youngster is pressured to (1) buy some marijuana, (2) leave the house against parental instructions, (3) smoke a cigarette, (4) let someone else copy his math homework answers, and (5) join in picking on someone. Ask for volunteers to role play each situation using appropriate assertive techniques. Stress the importance of assertive response, body posture, eye contact, and voice tone.

Decision-Making Skills

The purpose of this component is to teach children the proper method to use when confronted with a decision which might lead to the use of alcohol or other drugs. Consider the following from the Grade 9 to 12 portion of a curriculum.

GOAL:
The student will demonstrate the ability to use decision-making skills in making effective judgments.

OBJECTIVES:
The student will

- generate examples of situations in which personal decisions about drug use could affect the safety of themselves and others
- identify beliefs and principles concerning drugs
- evaluate past choices as a guide for future decision making

VOCABULARY:
Terms for the first objective above, for example, include

- responsible decisions
- consequences

ACTIVITIES:
Activities associated with the first objective above, for example, include

- Discuss with students that sometimes they must use their knowledge about drugs and their decision-making abilities to make responsible decisions about other people's drug use.
- Distribute a handout "For Safety's Sake." This exercise consists of four situations: (1) Your younger brother or sister comes home with a joint and asks what it is, (2) a friend at the end of a party is intoxicated and plans to drive home, (3) at a party you are hosting a couple of people become very intoxicated, get loud, and bother the rest of the people, and (4) at a party you are hosting, a friend lights up a joint and starts to pass it around. For each situation students are asked, "What would you do?" and "Why?" After completion of the handout, discuss the decisions made by the students. To encourage discussion, tell the students that there is no one correct answer. Explore the possible consequences if one followed the suggestions offered. Also, discuss the possible consequences that might result by not making responsible decisions.

CONCLUSIONS

As a teacher or a counselor, you can engage in many of the same prevention measures given earlier for parents.

A drug-abuse prevention curriculum consists of direct teaching methods (lectures, films, readings, field trips) and indirect teaching methods (role playing, group activities).

A grade-specific drug-abuse prevention curriculum begins in kindergarten and progresses with increasing complexity through the 12th grade. It includes learning components, goals, objectives, vocabulary terms, activities, and evaluations.

How Can I Tell If My Child Is Abusing Drugs?

The diagnosis of chemical dependence in adolescents can be difficult. They usually deny that they have a problem with alcohol or other drugs, and typically minimize their drug use and withhold information. It is important to realize that drug abuse is not the only cause of behavioral problems in adolescents. When drug abuse and behavioral problems coexist, however, it is highly likely that the bad behavior results from the drug abuse.

DEFINITION OF CHEMICAL DEPENDENCE

In 1956, the American Medical Association (AMA) declared alcoholism to be an illness, and in 1987 it extended its declaration to all drugs of abuse. Based on the AMA's statements, we arrived at the following definition of chemical dependence:

Chemical dependence is a chronic, progressive illness characterized by significant impairment that is directly associated with persistent and excessive use of a psychoactive substance. Impairment may involve medical, psychological, or social dysfunction.

This definition implicitly states several things:

- Chemical dependence is an illness; that is, a disease.
- It is chronic; that is, it takes place over a period of time.
- It is progressive; that is, it gets worse over time if it is not treated.
- It causes significant impairment from medical, psychological, or social dysfunction.

Medical dysfunction consists of such problems as alcoholic hepatitis (inflammation of the liver), pancreatitis (inflammation of the pancreas), bacterial endocarditis (infection of the heart valves), and AIDS (acquired immune deficiency syndrome). Psychological dysfunction includes anxiety, insomnia, depression, paranoia (an unwarranted feeling that others are out to get you), and psychosis (someone severely out of touch with reality). Social dysfunction includes problems with parents, friends, school, a job, and the police. The impairment must be associated with persistent and excessive use of a psychoactive substance.

The definition does not explain several things:

1. *Persistent is not defined.* Drug use every weekend is certainly persistent. One does not have to use drugs daily to be addicted. I like to ask medical students if a person who drinks only on weekends can be alcoholic. Many of the students are unsure. The correct answer is "of course one can." Consider a man who beats his wife every weekend when he is under the influence, and causes her to take the children and leave him. What if he has lost his job because of missing work on Monday mornings and he has multiple arrests on weekends for driving under the influence or for being drunk and disorderly. He is quite clearly alcoholic.

2. *"Excessive" is not defined.* It can be explained as the quantity of drug used in a persistent fashion that is sufficient to cause significant impairment in at least one of the three major areas of functioning—medical, psychological, social.

3. Withdrawal signs and symptoms on cessation of drug use may occur, but their occurrence is not required to diagnose chemical dependence.

ASSESSMENT

The key to the difficult process of diagnosing adolescent chemical dependence is a persistent, careful, and comprehensive investigation called an *assessment*. The assessment consists of gathering information about the adolescent's drug use, his medical status, including physical findings, laboratory findings, and drug screening results, and his psychosocial functioning.

Drug Use

As much information as possible should be gathered about the adolescent's drug use, including smoking history, alcohol history, and history of prescription and illicit drug use. Quite often, this information can be obtained from the adolescent's friends, ex-friends, girlfriend or boyfriend, ex-girlfriend or ex-boyfriend, or teacher. This, coupled with the information you may already have yourself, should prove very enlightening.

Keep in mind that many adolescents, especially the younger ones, tend to abuse substances that are not usually considered to be drugs. These substances may include glues, gasoline, paint thinners, mushrooms, Liquid Paper, and Scotchgard.

Drugs may also be used in unusual forms. For example, a 14-year-old female patient drank several ounces of Dr. Tischner's, an antiseptic high in alcohol content, every morning on the way to school. Her reasoning was very logical. She stated that she drank the Dr. Tischner's because she was too young to buy alcoholic beverages.

Medical Findings

The adolescent's family physician or pediatrician should be consulted for a physical examination, laboratory studies, and a drug screen.

Physical Examination

Adolescents, as a rule, exhibit few physical signs of drug addiction. Some of the more common ones follow:

• Untidiness in personal appearance and habits is common.
• Gastrointestinal problems occasionally occur because alcohol irritates the stomach wall.
• The eyes may be red and a chronic cough may be present due to marijuana abuse. Adolescent marijuana users usually wear sunglasses, even indoors, to cover up their red eyes.
• Pupillary constriction and constipation from opioid abuse may be present.
• Pupillary dilation, decreased appetite, and weight loss due to stimulant abuse may be present.
• Rhinitis (an inflammation of the nasal passages), nasal bleeding, sinus problems, nasal septal perforation (a hole in the cartilage between the right and the left sides of the nose), or nasal inhaler abuse may occur due to cocaine snorting.
• Suspiciousness, paranoia, and outright psychosis (being severely out of touch with reality) may result from amphetamine, cocaine, or phencyclidine abuse.
• Nystagmus (rapid, uncontrollable movements of the eyeballs), paranoid delusions, and delusions of superhuman strength may result from phencyclidine abuse. A delusion is a false idea that is believed to be true.
• Hallucinations and pupillary dilation may occur with hallucinogen abuse.
• Needle tracks on the arms, cellulitis (superficial infection of the skin), and abscesses from opioid injections may be present.

Addicts tend to wear long-sleeved shirts to cover up these signs, even in the summertime.
• Rashes around the nose or on the hands may be due to inhalant abuse.

Laboratory Findings

Abnormal laboratory findings due to drug abuse are seldom seen in adolescents. Occasionally one will have elevated liver enzymes in the blood, indicating liver damage as a result of alcoholic hepatitis. When local infection is present at injection sites, the white blood cell count may be elevated. In the presence of infectious diseases such as bacterial endocarditis (infection of heart valves), hepatitis B (viral infection of the liver), and AIDS (acquired immune deficiency syndrome) contracted by the use of dirty needles, specific laboratory signs will be present. A positive drug screen can be helpful.

Drug Screening

By itself, a positive drug screen does not make the diagnosis of drug addiction. It only proves that the adolescent has used the drug at least once. If, prior to the drug screen, he was adamant about never having used the drug, a positive result may have the effect of breaking through the denial, and forcing the adolescent to get honest about his drug use. A negative drug screen does not rule out drug addiction. For many drugs, it may only mean that a drug has not been used for the last two to three days. For other drugs, it may mean that they weren't screened for. Lysergic acid diethylamide (LSD) and MDMA (ecstasy) are two popular adolescent drugs that are not normally part of a routine drug screen. Ask your physician to add these two drugs to the routine drug screen.

Most drugs are water soluble. This means that they only accumulate in the parts of the body where the water is. Water constitutes about 60 percent of the body. It also means that they are rapidly excreted in the urine so that they disappear from the body within two to three days. In addition to the water, drugs that are fat soluble such as marijuana, benzodiazepines, and phencyclidine also distribute to the fatty tissues of the body where they are stored and released slowly after cessation of drug use. Heavy daily use of these kinds of drugs for an extended period of time can result in a positive drug screen up to four weeks after cessation of use.

Although a number of body fluids can be used for drug testing, the one most commonly used is urine. Collecting it is an easy, noninvasive procedure that does not require a hypodermic needle. It is easier to analyze urine than blood or other body fluids, and it can be refrigerated and stored while awaiting the testing procedure. Furthermore, drugs are usually found in higher concentrations in the urine than in other body fluids because of the concentrating ability of the kidneys.

Laboratory procedures for detecting drugs in bodily fluids are divided into *screening tests* and *confirmatory tests*. Screening tests are highly sensitive; that is, they seldom miss a drug when it is present above a preset cutoff level. However, they are not very specific; that is, they can incorrectly identify one drug as another, which is known as a *false positive* result. Screening tests have the advantage of being inexpensive. Because of the possibility that a result is falsely positive, all positive screening results must be subjected to a second, more expensive test, called a confirmatory test, which is highly specific and rarely, if ever, in error.

Urine drug screening has the disadvantage of not being quantitative, giving only a positive or a negative result. When quantitative results are desired, testing is usually done on blood. An example of this is the blood alcohol level (BAL) used to determine if an individual is legally drunk (0.1 gm/100 ml or greater in most states).

Adolescent drug abusers usually know of a number of ways to try to defeat the drug screening process. One common technique is to dilute their urine with water in an attempt to get the drug concentration below its cutoff level so that it cannot be detected; however, laboratories test urine samples for something called specific gravity, which is the density of a fluid relative to water. Dilution of urine with water produces a specific gravity outside of the normal range, indicating to the laboratory that the sample has been tampered with. Other methods adolescents use to try to defeat the process include substituting a non-drug-using person's urine for their own, and adulterating their own urine sample with vinegar, bleach, or lemon juice to interfere with the detecting process. Direct observation of the specimen collection should eliminate all of these possibilities.

Psychosocial Findings

With adolescents, the psychosocial assessment is usually much more helpful than the medical assessment. It should include information about:

Personal functioning

- Has his personal appearance and hygiene deteriorated?
- Does he lie, steal, and cheat?
- Does he have unexplained losses of money or possessions?
- Does he, for some unexplained reason, possess large sums of money?
- Does he wear clothing with drug-related slogans?
- Does he act secretively, for example, whispering on the telephone?
- Does he spend a lot of time in his room alone when at home?
- Does he spend a lot of time in the bathroom with the door locked?
- Has he had episodes of not remembering things he did or said—known as blackouts?
- Does he frequently use incense in his room?
- Does he say that he can quit using drugs anytime?
- Does his dress reflect an "offbeat" attitude?

- Does he seem to feel that the rest of the world is out of step?
- Is he preoccupied with drugs?
- Does he binge drink?
- Have you smelled alcohol on his breath?
- Has he tried to stop using drugs before and failed?
- Have you found drugs or drug paraphernalia in his room?
- Does he wear sunglasses, even in the house?
- Does he get into fights?
- Has he run away from home?
- Does he smoke (adolescents who smoke are at a higher risk for drug addiction than those who don't)?

Family relationships

- Have relationships with family members deteriorated?
- Is he verbally abusive?
- Is he generally rebellious?
- Does he seem to be involved in a lot of family conflict?
- Does he stay out late at night, refusing to give accurate information about his activities, or give flippant answers?
- Have siblings or relatives expressed concern about his behavior or drug use?
- Have items of value disappeared from the house?

Peer relationships

- Has he changed friends to a less desirable crowd?
- Are most or all of his friends drug users?
- Have his friends expressed concern about his behavior or drug use?
- Is he sexually promiscuous?

School functioning

- Have his grades declined?
- Does he skip school?
- Has he been in trouble with school authorities?

- Has he been suspended?
- Has he dropped out of school?
- Has a teacher or school counselor expressed concern about his behavior or drug use?

Leisure activities

- Has he stopped doing things he really used to enjoy?
- Does he seem to want just to "hang out" with friends all the time rather than participate in other activities?
- Is he overly interested in heavy rock music?

Employment problems

- Has he been fired from a job because of tardiness, missing work, or a bad attitude?
- Has a boss or fellow employee ever expressed concern about his behavior or drug use?

Legal problems

- Has he been in trouble with the law for driving under the influence, possession of alcohol, marijuana, or other controlled substances, drunk and disorderly behavior, or petty crimes?

Psychological functioning

- Does he seem to be on edge a lot?
- Does he seem angry all the time?
- Is he withdrawn or depressed?
- Does he seem to have a poor self-image?
- Does he undergo rapid mood changes?
- Is his behavior unpredictable?
- Does he seem to have lost the ability for goal-directed drives (amotivational syndrome)?
- Has he made suicide threats, gestures, or attempts?

Family History

Attention should be paid to the family history. Alcoholism, and probably other drug addictions, tend to run in families. A strong family history of addiction increases the likelihood that the adolescent is drug addicted.

MAKING THE DIAGNOSIS

Now, having gathered all of the information possible during the assessment, the next step is to use it to see if your child fits the definition of chemical dependence given earlier in this chapter. If the adolescent has significant medical problems, psychological problems, or social problems that appear to be coupled with persistent and excessive use of psychoactive substances, chemical dependence is highly likely. Steps to take in this case are outlined in the next chapter.

However, if significant medical problems, psychological problems, or social problems have not occurred, and the evidence indicates only experimental alcohol or other drug use, chemical dependence is less likely. In this case, the adolescent should sign a contract stating that he will enter treatment if drugs are used again, and he should be given another chance. If your child uses drugs again, despite having signed the contract, the possibility that he is really addicted increases in likelihood, and the steps outlined in the next chapter should be followed.

CONCLUSIONS

The diagnosis of chemical dependence in adolescents can be difficult. The key to diagnosis is the assessment—drug use, medical findings, drug screening, and psychosocial findings. Knowledge of family history of alcohol or other drug addictions can be helpful.

Adolescents who meet the definition given earlier in this chapter are considered to be chemically dependent and in need of treatment. Those who are using drugs but do not meet the definition should be required to sign a no-use contract and be given another chance. If they break their contract, however, they should also be admitted to a treatment program.

III

The Effects and Treatment of Drug and Alcohol Abuse

10

What Can I Do If My Child Is Abusing Drugs?

Having determined that it is likely that your child is addicted to alcohol or other drugs, the next step is to consult a professional. This can be initiated by placing a phone call to an adolescent alcohol and drug treatment facility. Many advertise on the radio or television, and all have listings in the yellow pages of the telephone directory. Alternatively, your physician or a friend may be able to recommend one. Place the call, and request an interview with an adolescent counselor or an addictionist—a physician who specializes in addictive disorders. The first interview is usually granted free of charge.

At the interview, present the information you have gathered in the assessment. Following this, the counselor or addictionist will interview your child and make a recommendation. They may determine that it is unlikely that your child has a drug problem and refer him to a psychologist to be evaluated for a behavioral disorder, or they may decide that it is highly likely that your child is addicted to drugs and recommend admission for treatment. If the information you provide is inadequate to make a diagnosis of drug addiction, but sufficient to suspect it, a short admission period for further evaluation may be recommended.

Now, suppose it has been determined that your child should be admitted for treatment. If he is willing to do so voluntarily, admission should take place immediately. If he is not willing to be admitted voluntarily, the problem becomes more difficult, but not impossible. Several options are available. Tough love and intervention are two useful concepts. Court-ordered treatment is another.

TOUGH LOVE

The purpose of *tough love* is to speed up the process of getting the adolescent to agree to be admitted for treatment. It consists of five steps: (1) open acceptance, (2) education, (3) support groups, (4) assigning responsibility, and (5) allowing the consequences.

1. *Open acceptance.* This concept consists of the parent openly accepting the drug-addicted adolescent as a person worthy of love. The love is unconditional. It is based on the adolescent's needs, not his bad behavior, which should not be condoned.

2. *Education.* Family members should learn as much as they can about drug addiction. As they learn about the hard facts of addiction, they will acquire the emotional detachment that is necessary to carry out the remaining steps of tough love.

3. *Support groups.* Family members should find local support groups, such as Al-Anon or Alateen, and should begin to attend the meetings. Interaction with others who have experienced, or are now experiencing, the same problems can be extremely helpful.

4. *Assigning responsibility.* In this step, the family quits making excuses for the adolescent's behaviors and actions, and no longer accepts rationalizations and excuses. The adolescent is expected to take responsibility for, and to be accountable for his own behavior.

5. *Allowing the consequences.* The adolescent is allowed to suffer the consequences of his or her behavior. For instance, you

shouldn't rush to bail your child out of jail when he gets arrested for a petty offense. Let him learn from the experience; it will do your child good. Eventually, he will come to see that he needs help. If not, an intervention can be done.

INTERVENTION

Intervention consists of two steps: preparing for a confrontation and the confrontation itself.

Preparing for the Confrontation

The purpose of direct confrontation is to convince adolescents of the effects of their destructive behavior and insist that they agree to enter treatment. During the confrontation, adolescents are told of the harmful effects of their behavior on themselves and on the people close to them. They are told of the consequences of continuing their drug-abusing lifestyle, and offered a way to avoid the consequences—treatment.

A family prepares for a confrontation by taking six steps: (1) consulting a professional, (2) choosing members of the team, (3) choosing the confrontation data, (4) choosing its time, (5) holding a practice confrontation, and (6) investigating treatment options.

1. *Consult a professional.* Every intervention team should have a drug abuse counselor or an addictionist to supervise the preparation and direct the actual confrontation. This should not be a difficult step since contact was made during the assessment phase.

2. *Choose members of the team.* Families should select members of the team on the basis of their close relationships with the adolescent and their willingness to participate in a confrontation.

Team members may be family members, friends, school teachers or counselors, and anyone who can play a positive role in the confrontation. Individuals who should be excluded include those whose psychological state is too fragile to withstand the emotional impact of the confrontation, anyone likely to berate the adolescent or preach moralistically, and family members too full of hate to perceive that drug addiction is an illness and that the drug-addicted person is in need of help.

3. *Choose the data.* With the help of the professional, each team member selects two or three examples of the adolescent's inappropriate behavior that has impacted negatively on them. These should be as detailed and as current as possible. It is imperative that team members focus on facts and observations rather than feelings and judgments. They should not use their information to try to humiliate the adolescent but to help him or her see the seriousness of the addictive behaviors. Angry, hostile remarks will only activate the adolescent's defense mechanisms.

4. *Choose the time.* A time for the confrontation should be chosen that is as convenient as possible for all members of the team. It should be when the adolescent is expected to be free of drugs, at least temporarily. If the adolescent is intoxicated at the scheduled confrontation time, it should be postponed. For some adolescents, the confrontation will have to be done in the morning before drug use begins.

5. *Hold a practice confrontation.* Members of the team should meet at least once, and preferably twice, to rehearse the confrontation. During these meetings, the professional plays the role of the adolescent, and team members practice giving their evidence in a detached, nonjudgmental manner. They should also practice how they will respond to the adolescent's manipulation, evasion, or anger.

6. *Investigate treatment options.* The last step is to investigate both inpatient and outpatient treatment options and the costs of each. Financial matters, such as insurance clearance, should be taken care of in advance so that, should the intervention be

successful, there will not be a delay in getting the adolescent into treatment.

The Confrontation

The intervention team assembles at the planned time. Once the adolescent arrives, the professional, who serves as the facilitator, speaks first, explaining to the adolescent why they have gathered and asking him to listen without speaking for a while. The adolescent is told that when everyone is finished speaking, he will have a turn. As rehearsed, each person then speaks directly to the adolescent, sharing facts, events, and personal reactions to his or her behavior, and explaining how it has adversely affected the speaker. Remember, an intervention is an act of love; members of the team should keep this in mind and act accordingly. Following the presentations, members then encourage the adolescent by telling him that help is available. The team should be prepared for the adolescent's response, which may be tearful acceptance, anger, hostility, counter-accusations, or bolting from the room.

If the adolescent agrees to enter treatment, he should not be allowed to bargain about when to go. Delay will only give him time to develop excuses about why he shouldn't go and allow for rationalization to explain the examples of inappropriate behavior that were presented in the confrontation. Once the group makes a decision, the adolescent should enter treatment without delay.

The Unsuccessful Intervention

If the intervention is unsuccessful, the family should attempt to get the adolescent to sign a contract agreeing that if drugs are used again he will enter treatment voluntarily. Family members should continue to work on their own recovery by attending Al-Anon and Alateen meetings. The process of tough love should continue. Eventually, the adolescent will see the need for help, or, because of difficulty with legal authorities, will have treatment mandated by a youth court judge in lieu of incarceration.

COURT ORDER

This is a reasonable alternative to an intervention. For younger adolescents, parents can present their findings from the assessment to a youth court judge. For older adolescents, who are out of the jurisdiction of the youth court, the same procedure can be used in many states, but through a chancery court judge. If the judge finds sufficient evidence of drug addiction, he or she will order the adolescent to be admitted to a treatment facility. The treatment professional can advise you of the status of the laws in your state.

CONCLUSIONS

If you feel your child is abusing alcohol or other drugs and he is not willing to accept help, the situation is not hopeless. You can institute tough love, organize an intervention, or get a court order in some states to have him committed to a treatment facility. If he appears only to be experimenting with alcohol or other drugs, you can attempt to get him to sign a contract agreeing that if he drinks or uses drugs again he will voluntarily enter a treatment program. If he refuses to sign a contract or if he continues drinking or using drugs he then should be court ordered to a treatment facility.

11

What Goes On in Treatment?

Once your child agrees to treatment, or is court-ordered to receive treatment, you must identify a program suitable for your particular adolescent. Generally, two options are available: *inpatient treatment* or *outpatient treatment*. Other less often used programs include half-way houses and therapeutic communities, known as *residential treatment*. The treatment professional is best qualified to advise you on which type of treatment is best suited for your child.

INPATIENT TREATMENT

Inpatient treatment takes place in an alcohol and drug unit of a general medical–surgical hospital or in a freestanding treatment facility. It is often referred to as *primary treatment*. The length of time of inpatient treatment varies, but may last four to six weeks.

Inpatient programs often have elaborate rules with some sort of behavioral privilege system. Patients may not be allowed to make or receive telephone calls or have visitors during the first week. Preaching, scolding, and lecturing are avoided. Adolescents resent it, and it is not effective. They have had enough of this at home without any positive effects. Because peer influence is a powerful force, it is used as much as possible. Patient government groups are important because they promote responsibility and accountability. They also build confidence and improve self-esteem. Group leaders are in charge of unit meetings and act as positive role models; unit secretaries record the minutes of meetings and post duties on bulletin boards; and other patients are elected to make coffee, clean lounges, act as buddies to new patients on the unit, and bring necessities for patients who do not yet have shopping privileges.

A good inpatient program uses a multifactorial approach to treatment which includes assessment, treatment plan development, rehabilitation, and discharge planning.

Assessment

Medical Assessment

A physician addictionist uses information provided by the family, as well as information obtained from his or her own physical examination, drug history, and psychosocial assessment, to verify the diagnosis and formulate a detoxification plan. Fortunately, most adolescents who abuse drugs do not have significant withdrawal symptoms upon cessation of drug use. However, because drug-addicted adolescents often minimize the magnitude of their drug use, they are all carefully observed for withdrawal symptoms by nursing personnel for 24 hours or longer.

Detoxification medication, if needed, is prescribed in a tapering dose over three to five days. Few adolescents need it. Medical problems, when present, are treated, and records from the patient's personal physician are requested when pertinent.

Psychological Assessment

Detailed psychological assessments are done early in treatment. Psychological assessment consists primarily of testing. Two commonly used tests are the Minnesota Multiphasic Personality Inventory (MMPI) and the Shipley Institute of Living Scale (SILS).

The MMPI has two sets of scales. The first set reflects the patient's degree of cooperation with the testing and indicates whether or not the other scale should be considered valid. The second set reflects his personality characteristics, as well as delusional, disorganized, or psychotic thinking.

The SILS is used to estimate verbal intelligence quotient (IQ). It also estimates cognitive quotient (CQ), which is an indication of the patient's ability to think and reason. The verbal IQ is usually minimally affected by years of drug abuse, but the CQ may be depressed, indicating some degree of loss of brain functioning. Repeat testing in three to four weeks will determine if this loss of intellectual functioning is reversible or permanent.

Social Assessment

This involves collecting data from the patient, family members, friends, teachers, and employers on the patient's level of social functioning. It includes his educational level, history of childhood abuse, legal history, childhood role models, family life, and a detailed life-long drug history.

Treatment Plan Development

Finally, a treatment plan is developed based on medical, psychological, and social assessments. Physicians and counselors list identified problems on a master problem list. Individual problems may be dealt with in treatment, may be noted and merely monitored, may be dealt with after treatment, or may require no action.

For each problem that is to be dealt with in treatment, a treatment plan that sets forth specific goals and objectives for resolving the problem is developed; it includes a projected time course for the resolution of a problem. For example, denial of drug addiction and poor coping skills are two common problems dealt with in treatment.

Each patient is assigned both a primary counselor to guide his day-to-day activities and a treatment team, which usually meets weekly, to discuss the adolescent's progress on each problem and to update the treatment plan.

Rehabilitation

Rehabilitation is the process of putting the treatment plan into action. It consists of (1) education, (2) group therapy, (3) life story, (4) individual therapy, (5) peer assessment, (6) recreational therapy, (7) coping skills and relaxation therapy, (8) support group attendance, and (9) spirituality.

Education

Despite significant experience with a variety of drugs, adolescents in general possess little factual information about them. To correct this, patients attend lectures or view films daily on such diverse subjects as the disease concept of drug addiction, the adverse effects of drugs on the body, psychological and social aspects of addiction to drugs, cross addiction, the various steps of Alcoholics Anonymous, the recovery process, and how to prevent relapse. They are also, from time to time, given specific reading assignments. In addition, regular school studies are continued.

Group Therapy

Group therapy involves from 10 to 15 adolescents and a group leader who is usually a certified alcohol and drug counselor. It is an opportunity for patients to deal with a variety of issues, aided by other group members. Group therapy helps patients identify feelings, see how their addiction has hurt themselves and others, and begin to see the need for change. It allows them to share feelings they have usually suppressed because of their drinking and drug using, and helps them identify the defense mechanisms they habitually use to hide their feelings. Group therapy helps young people discover who they are by listening to what others tell them about themselves.

Life Story

Early in treatment, adolescents are asked to write their life stories. A life story includes information about their childhood, family relationships, school, legal problems, treatment, and the future. Information about their childhood includes:

- strongest memories
- childhood friends
- games played
- happy times
- bad times (physical or sexual abuse, accidents, hospitalizations)
- sad times

Information about family relationships includes:

- members of the family and what each one is like
- how they get along with each member
- serious problems the family has had (deaths, suicide attempts, long hospital stays for physical or emotional problems)
- divorce in the family
- what the family does for fun
- what their parents do when they do something wrong (talk, hit, beat, ground)
- what their parents do when they do something well
- who makes the decisions in the family

Information about school includes:

- grades (elementary school, middle school, high school)
- behavior in the above schools (shy, class clown, arguments, fights)
- changes in grades after drug use started
- presence of reading or learning disabilities
- special education classes
- awards and accomplishments
- school suspensions
- appearances before principal or school counselor for discipline problems
- what his friends were like (elementary school, middle school, high school)

Information about legal problems includes:

- things done that were illegal, whether they were caught or not, such as shoplifting, stealing things to sell to get drug money, stealing money or cars
- arrests
- jailed or picked up by police
- selling drugs
- faking I.D. to get alcohol
- asking an adult to get alcohol for them

Information about treatment includes:

- things done to get placed in a treatment program
- feelings about being in the program
- what is being learned in the program

Information about the future includes:

- things about the adolescent that need to be changed
- things that are good about him
- plans for the future (after discharge)
- what he will be doing in a year

- if he thinks he will have more power over things when he is an adult

When the adolescent completes his life story, he shares it in group therapy with his peers.

Individual Therapy

Problems inappropriate for group therapy, or problems better dealt with on a one-to-one basis, are addressed in individual therapy. In addition, written as well as reading assignments are given and then discussed.

Peer Assessment

A special kind of group called peer assessment gives patients an opportunity to contribute constructively to the therapy of another adolescent who is having difficulty in treatment. Patients identify problem areas, such as dishonesty, defensive behavior, not participating in treatment, and other undesirable behaviors. One at a time, they get the opportunity to present their information to the problem patient. The patient is not allowed to respond defensively to these discussions. Quite often, peer pressure has a positive effect on improving attitude and behavior.

Recreational Therapy

Drug-addicted adolescents, as a rule, do not regularly exercise. Since adolescents have such high energy levels and are often bored, sufficient recreational activities must be available. Under supervision, patients are expected to participate daily in various structured physical activities. These activities may include basketball, volleyball, racquetball, walking or running, and swimming. Exercise improves depression, gives one a sense of well-being, and promotes a good night's sleep.

Coping Skills and Relaxation Therapy

Many drug addicted adolescents used drugs to relax and cope with stress. Now they have to learn to do these things without the use of drugs. Role-playing stressful situations to learn appropriate ways to handle them is a helpful tool. Patients learn to relax by means other than drugs—deep breathing, relaxation tapes, exercise, and other techniques.

Support Group Attendance

Attendance and participation in a 12-step support group such as Alcoholics Anonymous, Cocaine Anonymous, or Narcotics Anonymous is an important part of treatment. These meetings are held among patients in the treatment facility. Visits by program graduates exert a positive influence. They usually return to the facility periodically to conduct support group meetings or informal discussions. They are able to speak with credibility, and serve as living examples of adolescents in recovery. Attendance of support group meetings while in treatment is important because it introduces adolescents to the groups and familiarizes them with their operation and function. After discharge, patients are expected to continue attending support groups in their home towns for the rest of their lives. The disease of addiction never goes away.

Spirituality

Spirituality is an elusive concept; it is not religion. In the treatment of drug addiction, it is used in a much broader sense. It has been defined as being in contact with yourself, with those around you, and with a power greater than you. It is that which enables the growth of positive and creative development in a human being. It involves honesty, humility, humor, and hope. It is seeing the beauty that is all around us. Working within the

Alcoholics Anonymous program is a spiritual process, as is taking the time to stop and smell some flowers.

A spiritual identity crisis may ensue with the onset of the adolescent years. Preceding that time, young people grow up with and accept the values they receive from their homes, churches, and schools. Their acceptance of these values is automatic and comforting. Chemically dependent adolescents, however, are particularly bankrupt when it comes to spirituality. Sobriety, by contrast, brings a positive and creative lifestyle to counter their previous destructive and negative existence.

Typical Daily Activities Schedule

A typical daily activities schedule for accomplishing the rehabilitative process follows:

Morning

6:30–7:00	Wake up, hygiene, make beds
7:00–7:30	Breakfast
7:30–8:00	Devotional/community meeting
8:00–9:00	Lecture
9:00–9:30	Break
9:30–11:00	Group therapy
11:00–12:00	School (on the adolescent unit)

Afternoon

12:00–12:30	Lunch
12:30–1:30	Peer assessment
1:30–2:30	Coping skills/relaxation training
2:30–3:00	Break
3:00–4:00	Recreational therapy
4:00–5:00	School (on the adolescent unit)

Evening

5:00–5:30	Dinner
5:30–6:00	Free time

6:00–7:00   Study time
7:00–8:00   Support group attendance (AA, NA, CA)
8:00–9:30   Study time
9:30–10:30   Free time
10:30   Lights out

Discharge Planning

Assessing the needs adolescents are expected to have after discharge is called *discharge planning*. Part of discharge planning involves making a decision about whether the adolescent will be ready to go home or should be transferred to a less intense level of non-hospital treatment; that is, residential treatment. Discharge planning also includes decisions about aftercare meetings and support group attendance once the adolescent is discharged. The patient and the aftercare coordinator sign a contract spelling out the terms of aftercare.

OUTPATIENT TREATMENT

Typically lasting about ten weeks in length, outpatient treatment usually takes place in the evening for two to three hours, three to four times per week. Outpatient programs have fewer components than inpatient programs, and because patients have easier access to drugs, random urine drug screening is an integral part of an outpatient treatment program.

Day programs have recently become popular. These programs are very similar to inpatient programs in structure except that patients live at home and attend treatment during the day. Day programs are sometimes referred to as *partial hospitalization*. As in inpatient treatment, they attend school on the adolescent unit.

CHOOSING A TREATMENT PROGRAM

Inpatient and outpatient treatment each offer certain advantages and disadvantages. The advantages of inpatient treatment are a structured living environment, lack of access to drugs, more intense treatment, an impression on the patient of the gravity of the situation, and more integrated health care services.

The disadvantages of inpatient treatment include being more expensive, requiring the adolescent to be away from home, and absence from full-time school.

The advantages of outpatient treatment include the fact that it is less expensive, allows the adolescent to live at home, and allows him to continue going to school full-time.

The disadvantages of outpatient treatment are the lack of a structured living environment, more access to drugs, less intense treatment, less impression on the adolescent of the gravity of the situation, and less integrated health care services.

Making the Decision

Certain characteristics make a given adolescent more suitable for inpatient treatment. These are a deep, ingrained denial of drug addiction, physical addiction with an expected severe abstinence syndrome, significant medical problems, a failed attempt at outpatient treatment, and a dual diagnosis such as drug addiction plus a psychiatric disorder.

Certain situations dictate inpatient treatment. These are poor family support, having a drug-abusing parent at home, a distance greater than 40 to 50 miles from the nearest outpatient program, and court-ordered inpatient treatment.

In general, most adolescents do better in inpatient treatment; however, many insurance companies are now requiring a trial of outpatient treatment, with inpatient treatment being approved only if the adolescent fails outpatient treatment. The best advice is to follow the recommendation of the treatment professionals. They are in a much better position to make this decision than you are.

CONFIDENTIALITY IN TREATMENT

A federal statute mandates confidentiality in the treatment of drug addiction. Information in a patient's record can be disclosed only with the patient's written consent. If the patient is under 18 years of age, a parent or guardian must also give his or her written consent. Acknowledgment of the patient's presence in the treatment program also requires written consent. Patients must be informed at the time of admission, in writing, of the confidentiality requirement. The statute provides for criminal penalties for those who violate its provisions.

RESIDENTIAL TREATMENT

The two forms of residential treatment are *half-way houses* and *therapeutic communities*. Residential treatment is frequently referred to as *secondary treatment* or *extended treatment*.

Half-Way Houses

A half-way house is basically a transitional living situation between inpatient treatment and the return home. It is best suited for the adolescent who has not made sufficient progress in primary treatment to be ready to return home or for one with an unresolved family issue, such as a drug-abusing parent at home. In half-way houses, 10 to 20 patients live together with supervision, sharing responsibility for maintaining the house. They do their own grocery shopping, cook their own meals, do the housework, and wash their own clothes. They attend school during the day and can have a part-time job.

The half-way house provides a supportive, drug-free living environment, a low level of treatment, and a place to hold support group meetings. Patients also attend support group meetings in the local community. Half-way house treatment usually lasts two to six months.

Therapeutic Communities

A therapeutic community consists of a group of adolescents living together in one or more houses for the betterment of the whole. It may be the primary treatment or a secondary treatment for those not yet ready to return home from inpatient treatment. These programs are usually three months to two years in length. Their emphasis is on patient socialization. Some therapeutic communities require the adolescent to be separated from the outside world; others do not. Therapy is usually, but not always, strongly confrontational. Therapeutic communities usually have dormitory-style living, daily chores, family-style meals, and require members to help maintain the facility. They may offer educational and vocational training.

Many therapeutic communities have wilderness programs in which patients participate in such activities as camping, canoeing, and rapids rafting. Besides building self-confidence, these experiences show adolescents that it is possible to have fun without drugs. Varying levels of treatment are found from therapeutic community to therapeutic community. Traditional therapeutic communities rely heavily on paraprofessional staff, having only one or two professional counselors.

STEP WORK

While in treatment, adolescents usually complete the first five steps of Alcoholics Anonymous.*

*See p. 175 for the complete 12 steps.

Step 1. We admitted we were powerless over alcohol—
that our lives had become unmanageable

The purpose of Step 1 is to break through the adolescent's denial of the adverse consequences that substance abuse has caused him. He may be asked to

1. give three problems he now has that are related to drinking and using
2. give five examples of how drinking and using has caused him problems in the past
3. give two examples of negative consequences that await him if he continues to drink or use
4. give two ways he has tried to control his drinking or using and failed
5. check the examples of powerlessness and unmanageability which apply to him:

   • People tell me I drink or use drugs too much.
   • Others get mad at me when I drink or use drugs.
   • I've tried to stop drinking or using but started again.
   • I sometimes drink or use more than I planned.
   • I sometimes lie about my drinking and using drugs.
   • I have hidden alcohol or other drugs so I could use them alone or at a later date.
   • I have had memory loss after drinking or using.
   • I have tried to hurt myself when drinking or using.
   • I can drink or use more than I used to without feeling high.
   • My personality changes when I drink or use.

Step 2. Came to believe that a Power greater than
ourselves could restore us to sanity

Having admitted powerlessness in Step 1, Step 2 gives hope. Adolescents may be asked to

1. list three people who are more powerful than they and who can help them stay clean and sober
2. state who or what is their higher power
3. describe how their higher power can help them stay clean and sober
4. give one example of how things are getting better since they stopped drinking or using
5. check the "insane" things they did when drinking or using:
   - blamed others
   - lied to friends or family
   - manipulated others
   - made excuses
   - stole objects or money
   - got into fights or arguments
   - threatened others
   - made fools of others
   - played the victim
   - tried to commit suicide
   - traded sex for alcohol or other drugs

Step 3. Made a decision to turn our will and our lives over to the care of God *as we understood Him*

Having come to believe that their higher power can help them stay sober (Step 2), they take the action in Step 3.

"God as we understood Him" allows adolescents to choose their higher powers. For example, they may choose the treatment program, Alcoholics Anonymous, their AA sponsor, or God in the traditional sense.

Adolescents may be asked to

1. discuss why it is important for them to turn their will over to a higher power
2. give two examples of things they now worry about

3. give an example of a person they trust, at least a little bit
4. tell how it can help them to "turn it over" or to discuss a worry with a person they trust
5. give two examples of how they have tried to control their behavior and failed
6. give two examples of things they have yet to "turn over" and explain how and when they plan to do so
7. give two examples of things they have "turned over" in the past week

Step 4. Made a searching and fearless moral inventory of ourselves

The purpose of Step 4 is to help adolescents identify their personal characteristics, both those that are assets and those that are liabilities.

Assets are things like loyalty, punctuality, kindness, and patience. *Liabilities* in Alcoholics Anonymous are known as character defects: selfishness, alibis, dishonest thinking, pride, resentment, intolerance, impatience, envy, phoniness, procrastination, self-pity, having their feelings easily hurt, and fear.

Selfishness. For example, consider the child who needs a new pair of shoes. His alcoholic father puts it off until payday, but buys himself a fifth of liquor that night.

Alibis. An alibi is an excuse for drinking or using. Addicts call them reasons. "If my parents would just leave me alone, I wouldn't drink so much."

Dishonest thinking. "My dealer threatens to tell my mother if I don't keep buying drugs from him. It's not fair for her to be burdened by this knowledge, so I will have to keep on buying drugs."

Pride. This character defect causes chemically dependent adolescents to make excuses for their mistakes because they cannot admit to making them. It is sometimes called false pride in AA.

Resentment. A classmate makes better grades because he stays home at night and studies. The addict hates his guts.

Intolerance. This character defect is refusing to put up with beliefs, practices, customs, or habits that are different than your own.

Impatience. For example, getting angry because a parent keeps the adolescent waiting a few minutes—as if he never kept a parent waiting.

Envy. For example, a kid next door gets a new car. The addict can't understand why the other person got one and he didn't.

Phoniness. For example, buying his mother a much wanted present as evidence of his love. It is of course only a coincidence that he was about to get kicked out of the house because of substance abuse.

Procrastination. Addicted adolescents are always just about ready to wash the car, clean their room, or mow the grass. They are notorious for putting things off, "I'll do it tomorrow."

Self-pity. "Despite all the things I have done for you all, no one really appreciates me."

Feelings easily hurt. For example, walking down the street they speak to someone who is preoccupied and does not hear them. They get hurt and angry.

Fear. Addicts always fear the worst, whether it is real or imagined.

After listing the character defects that apply to them, they discuss in writing who their defects have affected adversely and how.

Step 5. Admitted to God, to ourselves, and to another human being the exact nature of our wrongs

Having admitted to themselves and to God how their character defects have adversely affected others, adolescents discuss the information with another person, as a sort of a verbal catharsis.

They will, in another step, make amends to those they have hurt except when to do so would injure them or others.

EMOTIONAL STAGES OF BEING DRUG FREE

The addicted adolescent's relationship with alcohol or other drugs is very important to him. As a result, many adolescents go through the grief process when they give them up. The process of grieving takes time. Adolescents usually complete the process because of the length of treatment programs. The grief process consists of seven stages: (1) denial, (2) bargaining, (3) anger, (4) guilt, (5) depression, (6) surrender, and (7) acceptance.

1. *Denial.* In this stage, adolescents do not believe that their relationship with drugs causes them problems, or else they think that they can handle their using in a responsible manner.

2. *Bargaining.* In this stage, adolescents are really saying, "Let's make a deal." The attempted deal may be with parents, friends, God, or themselves. One may say, for instance, "Dear God, If you will just get me out of this mess, I will never drink or use drugs again."

3. *Anger.* In this stage, adolescents experience anger about being forced to give up alcohol or other drugs. "Why me? Why do I have to have this disease? Other kids my age drink or use drugs and they don't have my problems."

4. *Guilt.* Guilt is a feeling that occurs when our behavior violates our values. In this stage, adolescents begin to feel bad about the thoughtless things they have done and the people they have hurt, especially those close to them such as family members and friends.

5. *Depression.* Depression is an obvious response to guilt. In this stage, adolescents begin to feel sad and hopeless. They understand that they have to give up drugs, but they just don't understand how they will be able to live without them.

6. *Surrender.* In this stage, adolescents admit they have a

problem. Surrender means knowing you can't solve your problems alone and having the courage to reach out for help.

7. *Acceptance.* Acceptance means that you own a problem; that it is yours. In this stage, adolescents accept the fact that they are responsible for their problems and that they are the only ones who can do anything about them. Acceptance is acknowledging that the relationship with drugs has to go and being willing to take the necessary steps to achieve sobriety.

CONCLUSIONS

Two treatment options are available for adolescents: inpatient and outpatient programs. Inpatient programs use a multifactorial approach to treatment—assessment, detoxification, treatment plan development, rehabilitation, and planning for discharge. The rehabilitation process consists of education, group therapy, individual therapy, life story, peer assessment, recreational therapy, coping skills development, and relaxation therapy.

Outpatient treatment is less intense than inpatient treatment. Urine drug screening is an important component.

Federal statute mandates confidentiality in treatment. Adolescents may go through the grief process when giving up drugs.

12

Do Young Women Have Special Issues?

Young women, like young men, are equally at risk for developing alcoholism, prescription drug addiction, and addiction to illicit drugs. Women, however, have the capacity to directly affect another human being—the unborn child—by their drug use.

ALCOHOL

In recent years, equality for women has included greater freedom to drink. As a result, heavy drinking is on the rise among young women. The number of women in the United States who drink alcohol has increased from 45 percent to 66 percent over the past 40 years. Surveys in the community indicate that 5 percent of women are heavy drinkers. Because society considers it less acceptable for a woman to be a heavy drinker than a man, a woman's drinking problem is often hidden or ignored by family, friends, school, and employer. This attitude delays or prevents alcoholic women from receiving help.

Ulcer surgery, gastrointestinal hemorrhage, fatty liver, hypertension, anemia, and malnutrition occur at significantly higher rates in alcoholic women than men. Women also seem to be more susceptible to the cirrhotic effects of alcohol. The death rate for alcoholic women is greater than the death rate of nonalcoholic women of the same age.

In the early days of ancient Rome, the drinking of wine by women was an offense punishable by death. This law, which prohibited alcohol use by women, was linked to the prohibition against adultery by women. Thus, the idea that drinking by women was associated with "loose" behavior was established early in Western culture. In contemporary American society, the woman who drinks in excess bears a triple stigma. First, she is included in society's negative attitude towards all alcoholics; second, she is subjected to the special disgust focused on the intoxicated woman; and third, the idea that drunkenness and sexual promiscuity are linked add to this burden of disapproval. As a result, solitary drinking by alcoholic women is more common than in alcoholic men. Thus, the female alcoholic is often referred to as the "hidden alcoholic." Society's negative attitude in general influences not only the behavior of the alcoholic woman herself, her family, and her friends, but it also affects the attitudes and expectations of those in the helping professions; that is, physicians, nurses, psychologists, and social workers.

Divorce rates for alcoholic women are much higher than for alcoholic men. Nonalcoholic wives are far more likely to remain with their alcoholic husbands than nonalcoholic husbands with their alcoholic wives.

When women drink at a rate comparable to that of men, their smaller size and smaller proportion of body fluid cause a higher blood alcohol level. Whereas men are inclined to snack while drinking, women are often dieting to stay thin so they drink on an empty stomach, resulting in quick absorption of alcohol into the bloodstream. Women who use oral contraceptives metabolize alcohol significantly more slowly than women not using this type of contraceptive. Furthermore, in the premenstrual phase, women absorb alcohol more quickly and completely than in the postmenstrual phase. Women tend to begin using alcohol at a later age than men do and they progress more rapidly into middle and late stage alcoholism, a phenomenon known as *telescoping*.

OTHER DRUGS

Women are particularly at risk for becoming dependent on prescription drugs. They make visits to physicians more frequently than men and tend to complain of nonspecific anxiety. As a result, they are often prescribed minor tranquilizers, such as diazepam (Valium), alprazolam (Xanax), or lorazepam (Ativan). They thus learn earlier in life that the use of chemicals is a quick and easy way to cope with stress. It is not as easy for many women to unwind with a few drinks in a bar as it is for men, so they are more likely to seek medical relief from stress.

Women are at risk for addiction to the same illicit drugs as men; however, some differences do exist. Female cocaine addicts, for example, have a greater incidence of major depression than men. Furthermore, abstinent women do not appear to recover from their depression as rapidly as men. Women tend to develop addiction to cocaine more rapidly than men.

FERTILITY

Psychoactive substances disrupt reproductive and gonadal function with sufficient magnitude in some women to cause infertility. Normal individuals may only experience subtle changes in sexual function. However, individuals with compromised reproductive function may exhibit infertility problems. The disruptive effects of these drugs are usually completely reversible with cessation of drug use.

DIAGNOSIS OF CHEMICAL DEPENDENCE

The information required to confirm a diagnosis of chemical dependence in young women is basically the same as that for young men. Women complain more often of a wide range of symptoms, including depression, anxiety, sleeplessness, lethargy, stomach problems, and injuries from accidents or physical abuse. Chemically dependent women have a higher incidence of infertility, postpartum depression, irregular menstrual cycles, and amenorrhea (failing to have menses). Female addicts are less likely than males to report difficulties with school, work, the law, or violent behavior. They are more inclined to report problems with their relationships and children as a result of substance abuse.

Additional questions specifically appropriate for young women include: (1) Do you ever carry an alcoholic beverage in your purse? (2) Does your drug use vary with your menstrual cycle? (3) Has your drinking or using had any effect on the regularity or quantity of your menstrual periods? (4) What effect do you think your drug abuse has had on your children? (5) Has there been physical violence in your home in the form of spouse abuse or child abuse?

TREATMENT ISSUES

Minority in Treatment

Women are proportionately a minority in most treatment programs, averaging about 20 percent of the patients. As a result, many chemically dependent young women find themselves in treatment programs designed for men. Women need to feel comfortable with themselves and are reluctant to discuss many of their problems in mixed company. Hence, all-women groups are important, especially in early recovery.

Alcoholic women are more likely than nonalcoholic women to have alcoholic husbands or boyfriends and to be at increased risk for domestic violence. Frequently, women addicts are incest survivors, victims of child or spouse abuse, rape victims, or daughters of alcoholic parents. To be most effective, a treatment program for chemically dependent women must address their practical needs, such as child care and job training.

Low Self-Esteem

Low self-esteem seems to be an important feature of all addiction, but particularly of women addicts. How a woman feels about herself depends on developmental, psychological, and societal factors. However, self-esteem for many is dependent on occupation. The lesser value assigned to tasks normally identified as women's work, and the lower salaries earned by women, are important factors in their self-esteem. Housekeeping and childcare in the United States are assigned little or no economic value. Most married women in the workforce still carry the major responsibility for the family cleaning, shopping, cooking, laundry, and childcare in addition to their outside employment. Both as a factor in her illness and her recovery, the importance of career should be explored individually with each chemically dependent young woman.

Childcare

Because responsibility for the care of children is usually part of the female role in American society, and because chemically dependent women are frequently separated or divorced, the female addict entering treatment is far more often the head of a single-parent family than is the chemically dependent male. As a result, childcare is a major need in the treatment of chemically dependent women. Women cannot benefit maximally from treatment if they are concerned about the welfare of their children. Feelings of guilt for being a "failure as a mother" may be a major problem.

Psychiatric Disorders

The most useful categorization of alcoholism is the distinction between *primary alcoholism* (no pre-existing emotional disorder) and *secondary alcoholism* (with a pre-existing emotional disorder). Most patients presenting for treatment are of the primary type. Among men, the most common form of secondary alcoholism is that associated with antisocial personality disorder. This is true of other drug addictions as well. In women, the most common primary type is that associated with depression.

Relationship to Others

A woman is often defined through her relationship to others. She is someone's daughter, someone's girlfriend, someone's wife, someone's mother, or even someone's ex-wife.

Life Structure

Structuring of one's life is important for all female addicts. If she goes back to the unstructured world of housework and child-care she runs a greater risk of relapse, especially if that is not her role preference. Educational goals should be explored, whether it is a high school equivalency diploma, a college degree, or a postgraduate degree. Trade schools should be explored and used as resources.

Sexuality

Most young people in treatment need to learn that relationships can be based on caring, and that they can hug each other and be otherwise physically affectionate without having sex. Some young women feel that they are helpless without men—that they need men to have their emotional needs met. Young girls in our society are taught how to tease and flirt to attract young men.

When alcohol or other drugs are combined with adolescent sexual development, destructive behavior usually ensues. For example, under the influence, boys and girls sometimes become sexually active. Some exchange sex for alcohol or other drugs. When young women high on chemical substances have sex, it is usually unplanned, often resulting in unplanned pregnancies, abortions, rape, violence, and feelings of guilt and shame. Many have experienced incest and child molestation. The treatment setting is often the first time some young women have trusted anyone enough to discuss sexual issues.

Eating Disorders

Young women can develop any psychiatric disorder. Two disorders, however, occur almost exclusively in young women: anorexia nervosa and bulimia. When present, these must be addressed.

Anorexia nervosa. This disorder is characterized by an intense fear of becoming obese, a disturbance of body image—feeling fat in spite of visual evidence to the contrary, weight loss of at least 24 percent of original weight, and a preoccupation with losing weight. Anorexics diet, exercise, and abuse diuretics and laxatives, even while family members and their physicians try to stop them. Death sometimes occurs from complications of starvation and malnutrition.

Bulimia. The main features of bulimia include recurrent binge episodes, awareness that the eating pattern is abnormal, fear of not being able to stop voluntarily, depressed mood following binges, use of diets, diuretics, cathartics, and self-induced vomiting. Bulimics tend to make their binging as inconspicuous as possible. They tend to binge on high-calorie foods. Overweight adolescent females who have to go to the bathroom after every meal (to induce vomiting) should raise suspicion.

THE PREGNANT ADDICT

The overwhelming majority of drug-abusing women are re-productively active. It is now abundantly clear that abuse of any mood-altering substance during pregnancy can cause serious maternal and fetal problems.

Many women addicts use more than one drug. The combination of alcohol, marijuana, cocaine, and nicotine is common. Evaluation of risk factors for the pregnant addict and her newborn must take into consideration all of these drugs.

Medical Problems

A 40 to 50 percent incidence of medical complications among drug-addicted women has been reported. These most frequently include anemia, endocarditis (infected heart valves), phlebitis (infected veins), cellulitis (infected skin), hepatitis, hypertension, urinary tract infection, and venereal disease. In addition, the intravenous drug user is at increased risk for contracting AIDS. Regardless of the route of drug administration, the economic necessities to support a drug addiction by illegal means through theft or prostitution, secondary malnutrition, and the associated unhealthy personal and family psychosocial environment further complicate maternal well being and prenatal care.

Obstetrical Concerns

Obstetrical concerns about the pregnant addict include low birth weight, preterm labor and birth, intrauterine infection, fetal distress in labor, and congenital abnormalities or birth defects. Opioid withdrawal symptoms in the adult include anxiety, increased respiratory and heart rates, nausea, vomiting, and abdominal cramps. If the cramps coincide with labor, they may be confused with premature contractions or abruptio placenta (premature separation of the placenta from the uterine wall).

THE FETUS

Since approximately 85 percent of drug-addicted women are in the child-bearing age, there is a corresponding increase in the number of infants at risk for a complicated prenatal and postnatal course, including congenital defects and withdrawal symptoms.

Congenital Defects

During the embryonic period, which encompasses the second to eighth week after conception, each organ system in the body undergoes a sensitive stage in its development during which adverse influences can cause the formation of congenital abnormalities (birth defects). During the fetal period, which extends from the embryonic period to delivery, the fetus has concluded new organ development and is, therefore, less likely to develop congenital malformations. Instead, adverse fetal effects are expressed as growth retardation, alteration of external genitalia, and brain defects. Behavioral and psychological disturbances may be expressed later in life by the affected child.

Alcohol

In 1748 a British physician noted that when gin became cheap, more mothers gave birth to babies that were physically defective or mentally retarded. In 1759, the London College of Physicians petitioned the British Parliament to reinstate taxes on gin, so that it would be less available and constitute less of a risk to pregnant women and their offspring. The *fetal alcohol syndrome* was identified in 1973. It consists of a combination of birth defects, including growth retardation, small head circumference, mild to moderate mental retardation (average IQ 68), and small eyes and facial deformities. In addition, there may be skeletal, joint, genital, rectal, renal, skin, or cardiac defects. To date, the full-blown fetal alcohol syndrome has been seen only in children of women who were very heavy drinkers during pregnancy.

Fetal alcohol syndrome, the leading preventable congenital birth defect, ranks third behind Down syndrome and spina bifida overall. Raising a physically and mentally handicapped child presents problems, particularly to a young mother who cannot cope with her own problems.

Less severe but significant birth defects, including some that are subtle, do occur in offspring of women drinking lesser amounts of alcohol. Neuropsychological testing of children of drinking mothers has found IQ scores lower than controls, as well as retarded development of concept formation and practical reasoning. Emotional instability, hyperactivity, distractibility, and short attention span were also significantly more prevalent in the children of drinking mothers. In addition, the risk of spontaneous abortion is increased. For every child born with fetal alcohol syndrome, as many as 10 others may be born with fetal alcohol effects.

A safe level of alcohol consumption has not been established. The best advice for pregnant women is to abstain completely from alcohol intake.

Benzodiazepines

Maternal benzodiazepine (e.g., Valium or related drugs) abuse may result in birth defects, including facial deformities, growth aberrations, and brain abnormalities. The facial features resemble those of fetal alcohol syndrome, although a greater focal involvement of the cranial nerves may occur. The infant at birth may appear to have a sullen and expressionless face and to have impairment of vitality.

Phenobarbital

Phenobarbital abuse has been associated with facial deformities as well as other congenital malformations.

Opioids

Common metabolic disturbances in the opioid-addicted neo-
nate include elevated bilirubin, low blood sugar, low calcium, and
low magnesium. Convulsions may occur, occasionally resulting in
death. Respiratory problems, such as aspiration pneumonia, also
occur, as do brain infarcts and hemorrhages. (An infarct is an area
of dead tissue which has resulted from inadequate blood supply.
A hemorrhage is an area of bleeding.) Prolonged exposure to
opioid drugs may cause irreversible damage to the infant's brain,
resulting in mental retardation.

Cocaine

Cocaine abuse can produce a variety of neonatal effects,
including growth retardation, small head circumference, and premature rupture of the mother's membranes. An increased incidence of abruptio placenta, prematurity, stillbirth, and spontaneous abortion occurs. Infants may have depressed interactive
behavior and impaired organizational abilities after birth, including increased tremulousness and startle response. Infants born to
cocaine-abusing mothers may suffer meconium aspiration leading
to brain damage or death. (Meconium is material produced by the
fetus's gastrointestinal tract while in utero.) There is also a tendency toward low birth weight and heart defects. Convulsions
may occur.

Nicotine

Nicotine causes a dose-related decrease in birth weight and
head circumference. Congenital defects may also occur. A permanent long-term effect on growth of infants born to mothers who
smoke has been documented. Early in life, infants of smoking

mothers appear to be less alert, and by age 7 hyperactivity may be present. By age 11, a decrease in general ability, most evident in reading comprehension and mathematics, may be present.

Marijuana

Marijuana appears to cause less fetal harm than many other drugs. No clear-cut visible birth defects have been demonstrated. Signs of brain excitation, including increased tremors, startles, hand-to-mouth activity, and reflexes may occur in marijuana-addicted neonates. Poor response to visual stimuli may also occur. A dose-related decrease in birth weight and head circumference has been documented. It is not clear if any long-term effects persist.

Phencyclidines

Virtually all phencyclidine (PCP) abusers are multiple drug users; hence, it has been difficult to determine the fetal effects of phencyclidine alone. Phencyclidine-addicted infants have sudden outbursts of agitation, rapid change in level of consciousness, increased lability, poor consolability, coarse arm flapping, tremors, and roving eye movements. Although they may have respiratory depression at birth, there does not seem to be an effect on weight or length.

Inhalants

Sniffing of volatile hydrocarbons containing toluene may result in a syndrome of prenatal and postnatal growth retardation, small brain, brain dysfunction, and cranial, limb, and renal abnormalities. Facial deformities occur.

Abstinence Syndromes

Physical dependence can develop in the fetus, as well as the mother. Symptoms of neonatal withdrawal are often present at birth, but may not reach a peak for 3 to 4 days of life. They may peak as late as 10 to 14 days after birth for some drugs, and can be severe. Specific withdrawal symptoms depend on the type of drug which was used.

CONCLUSIONS

Young women, like young men, are at risk for developing alcoholism, prescription drug addiction, and addiction to illicit drugs. Women drinkers tend to suffer more severe health consequences than men, and they develop full-blown alcoholism more rapidly.

Abuse of alcohol and other drugs can adversely affect fertility. During pregnancy it can cause serious problems in the mother and the baby. Birth defects are common in the offspring of substance-abusing women. Addiction in the mother can lead to serious withdrawal symptoms in both the mother and the child.

13

What Help Is Available for the Rest of the Family?

The effects of drug addiction on the user's family are profound. Members tend to function inappropriately in a codependent manner. Beattie defines a *codependent* as a person who lets another person's behavior—in this case, the addict—adversely affect him or her and who is obsessed with controlling the addict's behavior. It is estimated that there are 40 million people who are codependent for alcoholism. There are no statistics estimating how many people are codependent with addicts who use other drugs.

THE HEALTHY FAMILY

Most families are basically healthy, meaning that family members are usually happy, working, and contributing members of society. A healthy family, however, is not necessarily perfect. Members go through the illnesses, career crises, accidents, and losses that are a natural part of normal living. They suffer from all the usual stresses of raising children. Healthy families remain intact because they adjust to changes in a healthy manner. Curran has identified 15 traits of a healthy family.

1. *The healthy family communicates and listens.* Children in healthy families are able to observe open and honest communication between parents. Members are encouraged to share feelings, to think independently, and to support each other. They have the freedom to challenge each other in discussions because all members' opinions are valued. It is acceptable to disagree.

2. *Healthy family members affirm and support one another.* When mothers have careers outside of the home, family members accept additional responsibilities at home and support her efforts. As sons and daughters become busy with jobs and school, parents support their efforts. Responsibilities change and adjustments are made when parents' jobs require travel outside the community. One member's goals are as important as another's. Parents model self-esteem and set a positive mood within the family.

3. *The healthy family teaches respect for others.* Members of a healthy family respect each other's differences and opinions. Self-respect is taught. Each member is encouraged to develop strengths and talents. Respect for minority groups, other cultures, neighbors and their property is taught through role modeling.

4. *A healthy family develops a sense of trust.* Husband and wife role model trust toward each other and provide opportunities for the children to earn trust. The parents model dependability and thoughtfulness. When trust is broken, a healthy family uses the experience to teach that trust can be restored.

5. *The healthy family has a sense of play and humor.* All work and no play truly does make Jack a dull boy. Healthy families laugh together. Members don't take themselves too seriously. As a result, when the children are grown, they will have fond memories of growing up.

6. *A healthy family shares responsibility.* In a healthy family, children learn that their responsible actions create self-esteem. Family members recognize that responsible behavior includes recognizing the other members' emotional needs. The parents understand their children's capabilities and set their expectation levels accordingly. Recognition is given for accomplishments, and consequences are given for failure to act responsibly.

7. *A healthy family teaches a sense of right and wrong.* Parents agree on important values, and set clear, specific guidelines for their enforcement. They help the children distinguish between appropriate and inappropriate behavior. The children are expected to be responsible for their own moral behavior. The family has a strong moral base.

8. *Rituals and traditions abound in a healthy family.* A healthy family has rituals and traditions that are carried over from one generation to the next; it treasures its stories and its memories.

9. *A healthy family has a balance of interaction.* Children readily observe that parents are equal partners in family relationships. Separate coalitions of family members are not condoned. Work and activities are not routinely allowed to infringe on family activities.

10. *A healthy family has a shared religious core.* Healthy families integrate faith into their daily family life. Faith is passed on to the children in healthy ways. The religious core of the family nourishes and strengthens the family support system.

11. *Members of a healthy family respect each other's privacy.* Members of a healthy family respect each other's choice of friends, time alone, and personal tastes. Each family member is accepted and respected regardless of age, sex, talents, skills, or any other personal characteristic. The healthy family looks forward to their children reaching their teenage years when rules can be negotiated rather than set by the parents. Healthy families gradually let go of their children both physically and emotionally as they grow up and leave home.

12. *A healthy family values service to others.* Members of a healthy family demonstrate their value of service to others by such activities as car pooling, involvement in school functions, and service on community committees and task forces. The family accepts a simpler lifestyle so time is created for service to others. Volunteerism, however, is kept under control so that members have time for each other.

13. *Shared meals and conversation are valued.* Unfortunately, outside demands, such as team practices and committee meet-

ings, along with the ever-present television, are making unhealthy intrusions on family dinner table conversation. Mealtime is a time when family members can share achievements and frustrations, discuss their day, and teach values.

14. *The healthy family shares leisure time.* Balance is the key to sharing leisure time. To find balance, a healthy family prioritizes its activities, plans how it will use its time, and controls television watching. Members spend time with each other individually as well as within the family group.

15. *A healthy family admits to and seeks help with problems.* Healthy families don't seek perfection. They do admit their problems and seek help. They realize it's normal to have problems and teach their members coping skills and problem-solving strategies. Healthy families understand that having problems and solving them is a way to experience growth.

THE FAMILY WITH A DRUG-ADDICTED ADOLESCENT

A Family Disease

The family with a drug-addicted adolescent progressively becomes more and more dysfunctional. Members tend to develop their own unhealthy codependence in response to the stress of the situation. Family rules and family denial evolve, and members develop their own dysfunctional roles. Everyone whose life touches that of the drug addict is, in one way or another, adversely affected by the disease. Friends can drift away, a boss can fire the addict, the school system can expel him, but family members cannot so easily turn their backs on someone they love and someone for whom they are legally responsible. The only choice seems to be to do the best they can to adapt to the addict's illness and its effects on them. Unfortunately, there is no healthy way to adapt to drug addiction.

It is in the family environment that addicts find their greatest allies. Here, the people who suffer the most from the addict's behavior become the people who unwittingly nurture the addiction. The unhealthy relationships that develop follow a predictable pattern and cause drug addiction to be accurately labeled as a family disease.

Grieving the Loss

Drinking and other drug use tends to isolate adolescents from family events, from open communication, and from day-to-day interactions with family members. As a result, parents may feel they have lost a child and grieve the loss.

The grief process for parents usually involves six stages: (1) denial, (2) anger, (3) bargaining, (4) guilt, (5) depression, and (6) acceptance.

Denial

Unfortunately, parents are often caught up in the adolescent's denial, and develop a denial system of their own. *Enabling* plays a major role in parental denial. Enabling is a process whereby well-meaning parents unwittingly allow and even encourage irresponsible and self-destructive behavior in their children by shielding them from the consequences of their actions. They simply ignore the evidence of alcohol or other drug abuse. Because of parental denial, the average adolescent who is abusing drugs usually has been doing so for a year or more before the parents suspect and confront it. Typical statements made by parents in denial include:

- This is just a phase of rebellion. All teenagers go through this.
- He's just shy. That's why he avoids people.
- My child gets poor grades because he doesn't like school.
- He doesn't drink every day.
- He only drinks beer.
- I'd rather have him drinking at home than out using drugs.

- He will grow out of it. All he needs is more time.
- My child just picks the wrong friends. It's their fault.
- All I need to do is spend more time with him and everything will be all right.
- At least my child is not shooting heroin.
- He has so many pressures at school and with friends. I can understand why he feels the need to drink in order to unwind.
- My child just doesn't have enough willpower. He just needs to make a greater effort to stay away from drugs.

Van Cleave *et al.* have identified three important factors that contribute to the family's distorted perception of reality: (1) isolation, (2) emotional turmoil, and (3) centricity.

Isolation. It is unusual to find a family that talks to each other about an addicted member in its midst. Shame and embarrassment tend to build a wall of silence around each individual member and gradually cut off all but the most superficial communication. Family members tend to increase their isolation by cutting themselves off from outside friends and interests. The world of the family gradually narrows as each successive ring of involvement is peeled away, a phenomenon Talbott and Benson call the *target syndrome.*

Emotional turmoil. The family eventually becomes trapped in much of the emotional turmoil that afflicts the addicted member. They wrongfully feel guilty for causing the adolescent to use drugs and for having feelings of hate for someone they know they should love. They are ashamed and embarrassed by the addicted adolescent's actions, and they are angry at their own helplessness. They seldom share their feelings and emotions with each other. Instead, they suppress them and allow them to fester into a sense of despair.

Centricity. In the healthy family, no one person is always the center of attention. In the family with an addicted adolescent, that person is the primary focus of everyone's attention. The family is always on guard, trying to predict the unpredictable. Because of the stresses on individual family members they often internalize the rationalizations and projections of the addicted member, and like the addicted member, they tend to deny the addiction, even while paying an extraordinarily high price for it.

Anger

Once they are confronted again and again with the evidence—the discarded drug paraphernalia, the ever present Visine to clear the eyes, the mysterious capsules or powders, and the telephone calls from mysterious friends—parents eventually come to believe that what they have feared is true. In this stage, angry outbursts and arguments become commonplace.

Bargaining

In this stage, parents begin to bargain with their child. They make promises—the Florida vacation the child had wanted, a new car, a bigger allowance—if he will stop using drugs and running around with his "bad" friends.

Guilt

Bargaining having failed, parents turn their thoughts inward. Somehow, they come to feel that this problem must have been their fault. "What did we do wrong? How could we have raised him differently so that things would not have turned out so badly?"

Depression

Despite the attempts at bargaining, adolescents persist in keeping their drug-using friends, indulging in the same destructive behavior, isolating themselves from the family, and using drugs. Family rules continue to be broken and meaningful communication is nonexistent. For fear of what others will think, the parents are afraid to share their problem with friends, pastors, or counselors and, as a result, they become more and more isolated. The arguing, fighting, pleading, bargaining, and worrying takes its toll and they become increasingly depressed.

Acceptance

After sleepless nights, family fights, and hours of pleading and bargaining, parents eventually find it less exhausting and stressful simply to give up and accept the problem.

GETTING THE FAMILY WELL

Importance of Family Treatment

Most family members do not realize the extent to which their responses to the addicted adolescent—isolation, enabling, depression, anxiety, and even physical illness—have resulted from their own dysfunctional behavior. Therefore, it is imperative that the entire family go through a treatment process just like the adolescent does. Treatment of the family helps to set the groundwork for leading a normal, healthy life during the adolescent's recovery, not only for the adolescent but for the rest of the family as well. Addiction is truly a family disease.

Resources for the Family

Four useful treatment resources are available for the family: (1) family week, (2) family therapy, (3) codependent treatment, and (4) support groups. The treatment facility will advise you of what is available when your child is admitted.

Family Week

In some programs, family members join the adolescent the last week of treatment in the treatment facility. A typical family week would include interviews to determine each member's understanding of drug addiction. Presentations on such subjects as the disease concept of addiction, various steps of Al-Anon and Alateen, and information about healthy family functioning follow. Group therapy is an important part of family week.

Family Therapy

Family therapy involves group treatment of members of individual families, or group treatment of members of several families. Family therapy groups include the addicted adolescent. Sessions with members of several families are helpful for sharing experiences, for recognizing that the adolescent's problem is truly a problem that adversely affects every family member, and for breaking through family denial. Properly supervised confrontation between the adolescent and the other family members is helpful for releasing long-standing anger and resentment. Commonly, family therapy sessions are conducted weekly for up to six months after the adolescent has returned home.

Codependent Treatment

Treatment for family members or close friends who have been adversely affected by the adolescent's drug addiction is available in many treatment facilities. It is usually an outpatient program which follows family week. A typical codependency program lasts approximately four to six weeks and meets in the evening three times per week. Treatment consists of identifying and learning to deal with their own problem issues. They are introduced to a 12-step program for codependents which has been adapted from that of Alcoholics Anonymous, and they are expected to join support groups such as Al-Anon and Alateen. The treatment premise is that codependents can get well whether the addict does or not.

Support Groups (Al-Anon, Alateen)

Al-Anon is a fellowship of men and women whose lives have been adversely affected by an alcoholic family member or close friend. Its purpose is not to help the alcoholic stop drinking but to help those who have been affected by that drinking lead saner, happier lives. In essence, Al-Anon members admit they cannot control the drinking of others—that they are powerless to do anything about it. This allows them to begin dealing with their own lives more effectively.

Al-Anon members include those whose alcoholic is trying to stop drinking, has no intention of stopping, or has successfully quit. Members may be separated or divorced from an alcoholic, or the alcoholic may have long since died of his addiction. Al-Anon usually welcomes people whose lives have been adversely affected by nonalcoholic addicts as well.

Al-Anon developed as an outgrowth of Alcoholics Anonymous (AA) in the 1940s because family members in early AA groups learned from experience that they needed to apply the AA principles to their own affairs. As a result, they split from AA and formed their own groups.

Like AA, Al-Anon is compatible with all religions. It is a program that lets members perceive God in their own way. It lets people know that they are not alone, that others have the same fears and frustrations. It also gives them an opportunity to help others, an activity that gives them a great deal of personal satisfaction.

In 1957, a teenager whose parents were in AA and Al-Anon began a group for people his own age. It was called Alateen. Since that time, Alateen meetings, like AA and Al-Anon meetings, have become widespread.

THE FAMILY IN RECOVERY

The family in recovery gradually takes on certain characteristics:

- clear communication
- cooperation
- flexible roles and relationships
- open dependence on each other and acknowledgment of the freedom to talk about anything, to think any thoughts, and to ask for what each member wants and needs
- freedom to express any emotion and to pursue any goal
- empowerment rather than subservience
- enhancement of individual uniqueness
- use of authority to guide rather than to force compliance
- love, value, and respect for other members
- acceptance of personal and social responsibility
- the ability to use problems as challenges

In short, recovering families finally begin to resemble the healthy family described earlier in this chapter.

CONCLUSIONS

Most families are basically healthy. The effects of drug addiction on a family, however, can be profound. The family with a drug-abusing adolescent progressively becomes more and more dysfunctional.

Because parents are often caught up in a drug-addicted adolescent's denial, it is important for family members to also go through a treatment process. The family in recovery gradually takes on the characteristics of a healthy family.

14

What Happens When My Child Comes Home from Treatment?

It is naive to believe that when your child comes home from treatment all of your problems will be over. In the first place, it is a difficult task to raise a normal, nondrug-using adolescent. This won't change. In addition, family members will be learning to deal with resentments over past occurrences. At the same time it will be important for them to develop an understanding of the attitudes that can enhance or inhibit the returning member's recovery. Learning about recovery activities, such as aftercare and support groups, will also be important. Knowledge of the stages of recovery, partial recovery, and drugs—both illicit and prescription—that can lead to relapse can ease the process of re-entry for all concerned.

ATTITUDES IN RECOVERY

Attitudes are the result of life's experiences. One's attitudes may enhance recovery or inhibit it.

Attitudes That Enhance Recovery

Chemical dependence is a disease. Recovering adolescents with this attitude consider themselves to have an illness rather than being bad people. Thus, they are not bad people trying to become good, but rather, they are ill and trying to get well.

My disease is treatable. Like diabetes, there is no cure; however, chemical dependence is a treatable disease from which recovery is possible. Early recognition, diagnosis, and prevention have the same value for chemical dependence as they do for other treatable illnesses.

There is hope. Hope is the cornerstone of successful recovery. Hope leads to motivation for recovery.

The hurting can stop. When adolescents come to believe that there is a power greater than themselves, they can "turn it over" and stop hurting. Their siblings and parents can stop hurting, too. Believing in a higher power leads to hope.

Acceptance. Acceptance that one is an alcoholic or drug addict does not come easily to adolescents. Years of doing it their way have stood in the way of recovery. Early in recovery, adolescents may not fully believe that they can never drink or use again, and may attempt to return to those earlier days when substance abuse provided good feelings.

No one is responsible for my disease. Chemical dependence just happens. No one is responsible, not even the addict. Certainly, to become an alcoholic or drug addict was not a decision that was consciously made. I tell my adolescents in treatment that no one just woke up one morning and decided to be an alcoholic or drug addict when they grew up.

I am responsible for my own behavior. No one made the adolescent drink or use other drugs. No one, except the adolescent, will be responsible if he does so again. Excuses are accepted for what they are—false justifications for drinking or using. They are not valid reasons as the adolescent previously claimed.

Attitudes That Inhibit Recovery

Bad people drink or use drugs. Alcoholism affects the rich, the poor, the moral, and the immoral. Chemical dependence is an illness. Recovery is a process of being ill and trying to get well. *I can control my drinking or drug using.* Wrong! Alcoholics and drug addicts have lost the ability to control their drinking and using. Recovering adolescents cannot learn to drink socially or use drugs recreationally.

I can do it alone. Bill Wilson and Dr. Bob Smith, founders of Alcoholics Anonymous, were not able to do it by themselves. By joining together, they were able to stay sober. Isolation, a symptom of chemical dependence, does not lead to recovery.

Willpower is the answer. If willpower were the answer, chemical dependency would never have occurred in the first place. Recovery can only begin when one accepts that he is powerless over alcohol or other drugs.

Religion is the answer. While religion is good and is to be recommended, it will not keep one clean and dry. Alcoholism is a significant problem among Catholic priests. If religion were the answer, they would certainly not have a problem.

RECOVERY ACTIVITIES

Aftercare Meetings

Many treatment facilities have their own aftercare programs. Most facilities commonly conduct aftercare programs for a few months to two years following discharge. Usually, these consist of group meetings in the evenings twice weekly, and mainly deal with problems of reentry into society.

In addition to aftercare meetings, recovering adolescents are expected to attend two or three support group meetings—

Alcoholics Anonymous, Narcotics Anonymous, or Cocaine Anonymous—weekly in their community. Your child should be supported and encouraged to be involved in the activities spelled out in the aftercare contract. You cannot force him to participate in these activities. You are not responsible for your child's recovery; only he is. But you are responsible for your own recovery. Continued participation in Al-Anon and Alateen is a must.

Support Groups

A support group consists of recovering addicts who voluntarily meet regularly to help one another stay drug free. Alcoholics Anonymous is the oldest, largest, and best known of these organizations. Others such as Cocaine Anonymous and Narcotics Anonymous base their programs on AA concepts.

History of Alcoholics Anonymous

Alcoholics Anonymous had its beginning in Akron, Ohio in 1935 by two alcoholics: Bill Wilson, a stockbroker, and Dr. Bob Smith, a surgeon. Unable to achieve sobriety individually, they joined together to. stay sober through mutual support. Having achieved their own sobriety, they turned their attention to other alcoholics. They formulated the 12 steps of AA in 1938, and the book *Alcoholics Anonymous*, known as the "Big Book," was published in 1939.

Each autonomous AA group sponsors meetings that take place on a regular schedule one or more times a week. There are now over 48,000 AA groups in at least 92 countries. Alcoholics Anonymous has more than one million members in the United States alone.

*The Twelve Steps**

The 12 Steps of AA are a suggested model for the process of change and growth in recovery:

1. We admitted we were powerless over alcohol—that our lives had become unmanageable.
2. Came to believe that a Power greater than ourselves could restore us to sanity.
3. Made a decision to turn our will and our lives over to the care of God *as we understood Him.*
4. Made a searching and fearless moral inventory of ourselves.
5. Admitted to God, to ourselves, and to another human being the exact nature of our wrongs.
6. Were entirely ready to have God remove all these defects of character.
7. Humbly asked Him to remove our shortcomings.
8. Made a list of all persons we had harmed, and became willing to make amends to them all.
9. Made direct amends to such people wherever possible, except when to do so would injure them or others.
10. Continued to take personal inventory and when we were wrong promptly admitted it.
11. Sought through prayer and meditation to improve our conscious contact with God *as we understood Him,* praying only for knowledge of His will for us and the power to carry that out.

*The Twelve Steps and Twelve Traditions are reprinted with permission of Alcoholics Anonymous World Service, Inc. Permission to reprint this material does not mean that AA has reviewed or approved the contents of this publication, nor that AA agrees with the views expressed herein. AA is a program of recovery from alcohol *only*—use of the Twelve Steps in connection with programs and activities that are patterned after AA, but which address other problems, does not imply otherwise.

12. Having had a spiritual awakening as the result of these steps, we tried to carry this message to alcoholics, and to practice these principles in all our affairs.

Step 1 is admitting that one is an alcoholic and has lost control of his or her life. Having admitted powerlessness, steps 2 and 3 offer hope. AA members usually refer to "God as we understood him" as their "higher power."

Steps 4 and 5 involve self-examination. The purpose of this self-examination is not to dwell on the past, but to clear the slate and get a fresh start on recovery. Steps 6 and 7 allow God to change the alcoholic.

Steps 8, 9, and 10 have to do with accepting responsibility and being accountable. Step 11 is for continued spiritual growth. Step 12 involves helping alcoholics who are still drinking, such as accompanying them to meetings or helping them get medical care. This gives the "12-steppers" an improved sense of their own self-worth.

The fact that alcohol appears only in the first step underscores AA's contention that the main work in recovery is restructuring the alcoholic's life.

The Twelve Traditions

The 12 traditions assured that AA would not affiliate with other organizations, would espouse no cause other than helping alcoholics achieve sobriety, and would never accept outside funding or charge fees. Anonymity was insisted on at all levels of the organization to prevent individuals from using AA for personal gain. The 12 traditions are:

1. Our common welfare should come first; personal recovery depends on AA unity.
2. For our group's purpose, there is but one ultimate authority—a loving God as He may express Himself in

our group conscience. Our leaders are but trusted servants; they do not govern.

3. The only requirement for AA membership is a desire to stop drinking.

4. Each group should be autonomous except in matters affecting other groups or AA as a whole.

5. Each group has but one primary purpose—to carry its message to the alcoholic who still suffers.

6. An AA group ought never to endorse, finance, or lend the AA name to any related facility or outside enterprise, lest problems of money, property, and prestige divert us from our primary purpose.

7. Every AA group ought to be fully self-supporting, declining outside contributions.

8. Alcoholics Anonymous should remain forever nonprofessional, but our service centers may employ special workers.

9. AA, as such, ought never be organized; but we may create service boards or committees directly responsible to those they serve.

10. Alcoholics Anonymous has no opinion on outside issues; hence the AA name ought never be drawn into public controversy.

11. Our public relations policy is based on attraction rather than promotion; we need always maintain personal anonymity at the level of press, radio, and films.

12. Anonymity is the spiritual foundation of all our traditions, ever reminding us to place principles before personalities.

Philosophy of Alcoholics Anonymous

The single focus in AA is staying sober. Total abstinence is a basic tenet. Sobriety is considered to involve a happy, healthy way of life without alcohol. Alcoholics Anonymous considers alcoholism to be a disease, sort of an allergy to alcohol. The only requirement to be a member of AA is a desire to stop drinking. There are no membership cards or rolls; one is a member if one says so. Membership is free, supported only by voluntary contributions from its members.

Alcoholics Anonymous slogans for newly sober members are purposefully simple, direct, and catchy. For example, the slogan "One day at a time" means to focus on not drinking today.

The AA Sponsor

Veteran AA members with at least one year of sobriety can serve as sponsors for new members. Sponsors offer guidance, support, and confrontation if needed. Sponsors serve as powerful role models. They have what new members seek—sobriety.

Veteran AA members become a new member's sponsor by mutual agreement. Traditionally, to avoid intimate relationships, sponsors are of the same sex as the newcomer.

The AA Meeting

There are two basic types of AA meetings: open ones and closed ones. Anyone can attend open meetings, whether or not he has an alcohol problem. Only AA members and those wishing to stop drinking can attend closed meetings. Closed meetings function more or less as leaderless support groups.

Although they vary somewhat, AA meetings generally follow similar formats:

• They begin with a moment of silence.

• Next, members recite the serenity prayer, which has a message for everyone:

> God grant me the serenity to accept the things I cannot change,
> the courage to change the things I can,
> and the wisdom to know the difference.

• Next, an assigned member reads a passage about what AA is and is not.

Alcoholics Anonymous is a fellowship of men and women who share their experience, strength, and hope with each other that they may solve their common problem and help others to recover from alcoholism.

The only requirement for membership is a desire to stop drinking. There are no dues or fees for AA membership; we are self-supporting through our own contributions. AA is not allied with any sect, denomination, politics, organization, or institution; does not wish to engage in any controversy; neither endorses nor opposes any causes. Our primary purpose is to stay sober and help other alcoholics to achieve sobriety.

• This is followed by another member reading from the first part of Chapter 5 of *Alcoholics Anonymous*, also known as the Big Book, about how AA works.

Our stories disclose in a general way what we used to be like, what happened, and what we are like now. If you have decided you want what we have and are willing to go to any length to get it—then you are ready to take certain steps.

At some of these we balked. We thought we could find an easier, softer way. But we could not. With all the earnestness at our command, we beg of you to be fearless and thorough from the very start. Some of us have tried to hold on to our old ideas and the result was nil until we let go absolutely.

Remember that we deal with alcohol—cunning, baffling, powerful! Without help it is too much for us. But there is One who has all power—that One is God. May you find Him now!

Half measures availed us nothing. We stood at the turning point. We asked His protection and care with complete abandon.

Here are the steps we took, which are suggested as a program of recovery.

• The Twelve Suggested Steps of AA are then read. Afterwards, the reading continues from Chapter 5 of the Big Book.

Many of us exclaimed, "What an order! I can't go through with it." Do not be discouraged. No one among us has been able to maintain anything like perfect adherence to these principles. We are not saints. The point is, that we are willing to grow along spiritual lines. The principles we have set down are guides to progress. We claim spiritual progress rather than spiritual perfection.

Our description of the alcoholic, the chapter to the agnostic, and our personal adventures before and after make clear three pertinent ideas: (a) That we were alcoholic and could not manage our own lives. (b) That probably no human power could have relieved our alcoholism. (c) That God could and would if He were sought.

• After this, the major part of the meeting, the program, takes place. It may take one of several forms. In a Big Book program, members read selections of *Alcoholics Anonymous*. After each section, members discuss how the particular passage relates to their experience. In a step program, members discuss the various 12 steps. In a topic program, members discuss a topic such as gratitude, resentment, or acceptance. Each member relates what the topic means to him. A topic is usually chosen by the chairperson prior to the meetings. Some programs involve members discussing personal problems related to recovery. In speakers meetings, recovering alcoholics, usually from other AA groups, tell their "drunkalogues," which are accounts of the speaker's problems with alcohol and their process of recovery.

THE RECOVERY PROCESS

Recovery is a process in which the medical, psychological, and social damage caused by drug addiction is healed. Abstinence is the cornerstone of recovery. Recovery is an individual process. No two people recover at exactly the same rate. It is a lifelong process.

Stages in the Recovery Process

Gorski divides the recovery process into six stages:

1. *Pretreatment.* Addicts finally admit they are powerless over alcohol and other drugs. Most often, this stage occurs in the treatment program before returning home.

2. *Stabilization.* Addicts recover from acute drug withdrawal and health problems. They regain control of their thought processes, emotions, judgment, and behavior. This stage occurs, or at least begins, in the treatment program.

3. *Early recovery.* Addicts accept the disease of addiction and begin to learn to function without psychoactive substances. This stage relies heavily on a structured recovery program, such as that spelled out in the aftercare contract. It begins when the addict returns home from treatment. This stage may be difficult for some recovering addicts because of the postacute abstinence syndrome.

The adolescent learns to tolerate anxiety, solve the little problems of life, and anticipate the urge to use drugs when things get rough, or wonderful. The family learns to set limits. Family members learn to cooperate, work, and play together without conflicts erupting into rage. The family learns that mistrust is normal at this stage but that it will get better.

4. *Middle recovery.* In this period, the primary goal is to change lifestyles; it is less structured than early recovery. Resisting temptation to substitute other addictions, such as gambling, is an important issue in this stage.

The adolescent and the family are committed to healthy, drug-free activities. Everyone is learning to be more comfortable with dysphoric feelings and conflict. The adolescent learns to balance the demands of life—school, work, friends, and parents. He learns to manage self-doubt and to plan ahead to prevent problems from occurring. The adolescent learns to deal with boredom and the need for thrills. He or she begins to focus on the future, including college and leaving home. Parents begin to refocus on their marriage, deal with the issue of their child leaving home, and keep active in their self-help groups.

5. *Late recovery.* The primary goal of this stage is to develop self-esteem, the capacity for healthy intimacy, and the ability to live happily and productively. One evaluates personal beliefs, beliefs about one's self and others, self-defeating patterns of living, intimacy and relationship skills and, if needed, restructures them.

In this stage, parents learn to deal with their teenager shifting from the role of child to young adult.

6. *Maintenance.* The primary goal of this stage is for addicts to stay sober and maintain an effective recovery program. This involves identifying warning signs of relapse, daily problem solving, maintaining honesty, and living productively. In this stage, the adolescent is emerging into young adulthood. He, along with other family members, are maintaining a dynamic recovery plan and know how to prevent relapse.

Recovery is a lifelong process. The disease of drug addiction never goes away.

Partial Recovery

The recovery process does not follow a straight path. Recovering addicts reach and overcome plateaus, slip backwards occasionally, but usually move on to achieve long-term, comfortable sobriety. Others, however, do not make it all the way through the recovery process and relapse. Gorski describes a concept called *partial recovery* that begins when a recovering addict confronts a recovery task he believes to be insurmountable. He becomes stuck at this level of the recovery process. Instead of taking the necessary steps to overcome their failure and progress, many simply deny that anything is wrong. With help, many of these people overcome their denial and again begin to make progress. Others go on to relapse. The Big Book calls failure to progress in recovery "half-measures."

CONTROLLED DRINKING

In 1976, a study by the Rand Corporation reported that a significant number of alcoholics could learn to drink socially. Since then, however, that study has fallen into disrepute, and several other studies have not borne out its findings. Even if a small percentage of alcoholics could become social drinkers, there is no way to identify which ones they would be. An alcoholic trying to drink socially would be like playing Russian roulette; abstinence remains the only sure way to control alcoholism.

DRUGS THAT MAY BE HAZARDOUS TO RECOVERY

Many drugs, whether legal, prescription, over-the-counter, or illicit can be hazardous to recovery. Recovering adolescents should be especially leery of

- alcoholic beverages
- medications containing alcohol
- sedative-hypnotics (tranquilizers and sleeping pills)
- opioids (narcotic pain and cough medications)
- stimulants (including diet pills)
- all illicit drugs

Relapse has also occurred from the use of seemingly harmless drugs:

- antihistamines (Atarax, Benadryl, Phenergan, Tavist, Vistaril)
- decongestants (phenylephrine, phenylpropanolamine, pseudoephedrine)
- muscle relaxants (Flexeril, Norflex, Robaxin, Soma)
- antidepressants (Elavil, Ludiomil, Norpramin, Desyrel, Sinequan, Tofranil)

Classical antihistamines and decongestants are common ingredients in cold, cough, and allergy preparations. As a general rule, these should be avoided. However, newer, nonsedating antihistamines such as Seldane, Hismanal, or Claritin are much safer for recovering people. Muscle relaxant abuse is not uncommon. Antidepressants should be taken only when absolutely necessary, and then only under the care of a physician knowledgeable about drug abuse.

Although antihistamines, decongestants, muscle relaxants, and antidepressants are not physically addicting, they are sometimes abused for the mood-altering effects they produce.

RATIONAL USE OF MEDICATIONS

Recovering individuals undergoing surgery can have narcotic pain medication and, in fact, can have just as much of it as anyone else; however, some special rules apply. When possible, adolescents should stay in the hospital a few extra days if it means they can go home narcotic-free. In many cases, over-the-counter nonsteroidal drugs like Advil or Nuprin or their prescription counterparts, Motrin and Toradol, are effective substitutes for narcotics after returning home. If narcotic pain medication must be taken at home, the adolescent should not be given access to it. A family member or friend who is reliable should dispense it as prescribed. It should be taken for as short a period of time as possible, and as soon as the adolescent is able, he should temporarily increase attendance at support groups. The same rules apply for dental procedures requiring pain medication or other medical procedures requiring psychoactive substances.

PHARMACOLOGICAL APPROACHES

Several pharmacological approaches are available to help support recovery. They have, however, found little use in adolescents. Nevertheless, a little knowledge of two of these may be helpful.

Disulfiram. Disulfiram (Antabuse) is occasionally prescribed to help support alcoholics in recovery. It is a safe medication with relatively few side effects. Recovering alcoholics take it daily with knowledge that if they drink while taking the medication, they will become very ill, experiencing nausea, vomiting, and flushing. This knowledge is supposed to keep alcoholics from drinking. Its long-term effectiveness is controversial.

Naltrexone. Naltrexone (Trexan) is occasionally prescribed to help support recovery in narcotic addicts. It works by interacting with the opioid receptors so that, if the addict uses a narcotic, it cannot reach the receptors to cause its effect. By interacting with the receptors, it also diminishes opioid craving. The long-term effectiveness of Trexan is also controversial.

FAMILIES RECOVER TOO

Like adolescents, families too must go through a recovery process. If family members completed a family treatment program and have been going to family support groups, hopefully the adolescent and other family members will arrive at the same place at the same time. Even in the ideal situation, though, relationships need to be rebuilt and trust regained. Both take time. The emotional pains of the past don't die easily. With both adolescent and other family members working their program, however, family recovery is highly likely.

CONCLUSIONS

Alcoholics Anonymous is the oldest, largest, and best known of the recovery support groups. Its single focus is on staying sober. Other support groups include Cocaine Anonymous and Narcotics Anonymous.

Recovery is a process in which the medical, psychological, and social damage caused by substance abuse is healed. It consists of six steps, with the last one being the maintenance stage.

Controlled drinking or drug using by recovering addicts is a dangerous concept. Total abstinence is the only way.

Families too must go through a recovery process.

15

What If Drugs Are Used Again?

The ever-present risk of relapse can be a major parental concern. Understanding the relapse process, factors contributing to relapse, how the risk of relapse can be reduced, and what to do should relapse occur can help ease concerns.

THE RELAPSE PROCESS

Relapse, like recovery, is also a process. The actual act of returning to drinking or drug use is preceded by changes in behavior, attitude, feelings or emotions, and thinking. Symptoms of the relapse process, prior to the drinking or using episode, include fatigue, dishonesty with self and others, impatience, argumentativeness (a need to be right), depression, frustration, self-pity, cockiness, complacency, expecting too much from others, letting up on recovery disciplines, wanting too much, omnipotence (having all the answers), and an "it can't happen to me" attitude. In Alcoholics Anonymous, this is spoken of as "stinking thinking," "building up to a drink," and "dry drunk."

Several steps, outlined by Gorski and Miller, generally lead up to the drug-using act itself.

1. *Return of denial.* The relapse process begins with the return of denial. Addicts begin to feel that maybe they don't need all this "recovery stuff." They deny these feelings, even to themselves.

2. *Avoidance and defensive behaviors.* Support group attendance begins to be a chore, and attendance begins to lapse. They make excuses for missing meetings and come to believe that a daily recovery program is unnecessary. A lot of the old behavior (when they were using drugs) returns. They begin judging the other guy's recovery program instead of taking a good look at their own.

3. *Crisis building.* Isolation from others begins. They tend to develop tunnel vision—seeing only one small part of life rather than the whole picture. This creates the illusion that all is going well when it really is not. They begin to make plans based more on wishful than realistic thinking, and as a result things begin to go wrong in their lives. Periods of minor depression occur.

4. *Immobilization.* Daydreaming and wishful thinking increase, and they frequently use the expression "if only" in conversations. They have a wish to be happy, without identifying what it would take to be happy. They want to feel better without doing anything to make themselves better.

5. *Confusion and overreaction.* They become irritable and overreact to small things. They are easily angered, becoming frustrated and resentful for no apparent reason.

6. *Depression.* Depression increases in intensity, and, at times, they think of drinking or using drugs, or even suicide. They may seem unable to take action and have irregular eating and sleeping patterns.

7. *Behavioral loss of control.* Their lives become more chaotic. They fail to see the importance of attending support group meetings. Other things seem to be more important to them, and they develop an "I don't care" attitude. They become dissatisfied with life, which seems to have become unmanageable since they got sober. They begin to feel that they might as well starting drinking or using drugs again.

8. *Recognition of loss of control.* Isolation increases in magnitude, and they feel sorry for themselves, often using self-pity to

get sympathy from family members and friends. They begin to feel that they can drink or use drugs in a social manner without having all the problems they had before. They feel overwhelmed by their inability to take action to resolve their problems.

9. *Option reduction.* They begin to believe that help is not available to them. They stop attending support group meetings altogether and feel lonely, frustrated, and angry. They have more and more difficulty controlling their thoughts, emotions, and judgment.

10. *The acute relapse episode.* Finally, the relapse episode occurs: they take a drink or use a drug. They feel shame and guilt and make attempts to hide the fact that relapse has occurred. The alcohol or drug use rapidly progresses until in a very short period of time, usually a few weeks, their use is back to the level where it was at the time they went into treatment. All of the problems that accompanied their prior drug use reappear.

FACTORS CONTRIBUTING TO RELAPSE

Talbott has identified 13 factors that contribute to relapse:

1. *Failure to understand and accept drug addiction as a disease.* This is the fundamental factor that can precipitate relapse. Addicts who do not believe addiction to be a disease see no need for a recovery program. They feel that they can stay "clean and dry" by willpower alone.

2. *Denial of loss of control.* Addicts who don't believe in loss of control feel that they can use drugs as long as they do so carefully. They tend to do the same old things and expect different results.

3. *Dishonesty.* For addicts, dishonesty usually means distorting reality and concealing emotions, including those related to drug use. The popular AA slogan, "It's a program of honesty," indicates that dishonesty and recovery are not compatible.

4. *The dysfunctional family.* A healthy family can contribute immensely to recovery; however, a dysfunctional family can con-

tribute to relapse, just as it contributed to the progression of the disease.

5. *Lack of a spiritual program.* The lack of a spiritual program leads addicts to believe that no source of strength, other than themselves, is available to them. The concept of a higher power loses its importance in their recovery.

6. *Stress.* Drugs, for many, were a way of handling stress. Many times stress in recovery will initiate the return of drug craving. The acronym HALT stands for *h*ungry, *a*ngry, *l*onely, or *t*ired, all factors which in excess can lead to relapse. Self-pity, in the same way, can lead to relapse.

7. *Isolation.* Withdrawal from relationships in recovery can lead to a relapse. Too much time to think about one's self can lead to feeling hopeless, different, and worthless. Rather than withdrawing from relationships because of conflicts, addicts must learn to resolve conflicts and maintain relationships.

8. *Cross-addiction.* Having once been addicted to a psychoactive substance, recovering addicts can never again use any psychoactive substance without a serious risk of becoming addicted to it, or its use leading back to use of their original drug of choice. In addition, the use of mood-altering, over-the-counter, or prescription medications for colds, cough, allergy, pain, anxiety, or surgical procedures can also lead to a relapse.

9. *Holiday syndrome.* The risk of relapse is high at special times of the year, such as Thanksgiving, Christmas, or birthdays, when memories of the past surface and increase the pain of the present. In addition, these are high-risk times even when things are going exceptionally well. The "need to celebrate" can also lead to relapse. During these times, recovering addicts should go to additional support group meetings, call their sponsors, and work their 12-step programs.

10. *Postacute abstinence syndrome.* Many people think that withdrawal from drugs involves only the acute process, which lasts 4 to 5 days. However, a lower intensity of withdrawal symptoms, called the *postacute abstinence syndrome*, occurs. This syn-

drome may last for a few weeks to months and is a major contributing factor to relapse.

11. *Overconfidence.* When first in recovery, life's problems at last seem to be manageable. Addicts can easily come to believe that things will continue to go well regardless of what they do and discard their sense of humility and the need for a higher power. This overconfidence leads them to believe that they can once again drink or use drugs in a social manner, without experiencing all of the problems that drinking and drug using caused them in the past.

12. *Returning to drinking/drug-using friends and old habits.* Recovering addicts may come to believe that they can return to old drug-using friends and places without the temptation to drink or use again. The next step is for them to come to believe that they can also drink or use successfully. The AA slogan "Avoid old faces and old places" is borne of wisdom.

13. *Guilt over the past.* Dwelling on past indiscretions that led to the harm of others can lead to relapse. To achieve sobriety, recovering addicts must take a moral inventory of whom they have harmed (AA step 4) and make amends for their past actions (AA step 9), thus acknowledging the past and making peace with it.

PREVENTING RELAPSE

Relapse is not inevitable. It can be prevented. The aftercare contract spells out the basic steps. The core of any good recovery program is regular support group attendance and participation, along with the effective use of a sponsor. Adolescents need to "work their programs" one day at a time, every day, for the rest of their lives. When they are not in recovery, they are in danger of relapse. They should be familiar with the relapse process, as well as the factors that contribute to relapse. Being knowledgeable yourself about the steps in the relapse process will allow you to help your child identify his own relapse process should it begin.

Knowing the factors that contribute to relapse will allow you to support your child in avoiding them.

WHAT TO DO WHEN RELAPSE OCCURS

A relapse process is considered to be complete when use of the psychoactive substance takes place. When adolescents recognize this act as a serious one that has potentially devastating effects, some manage to get back in to the recovery process and do well. Such a brief encounter with drugs, followed by a return to recovery is sometimes referred to as a "slip." Others, however, continue to use drugs and very rapidly return to the unfortunate state of affairs that existed before treatment. For addicts who regret relapsing and wish to be back in recovery, several steps recommended by Talbott should be taken:

1. *Call their sponsors.* Sponsors are recovering people with a successful record in recovery. Many of them have been through the relapse process themselves and can give good advice. At this point, their support is very valuable.

2. *Call support group friends.* Addicts who have relapsed should call some of their support group friends immediately and report the relapse. Their support should be requested.

3. *Go to a support group meeting.* Addicts who have relapsed should go to their support groups as soon as possible and discuss the relapse. They should continue to go at least daily for a period of time and work on the cause of the relapse.

4. *Discuss the relapse with their physician.* If addicts have physicians that are knowledgeable about addiction, and who have been active in supporting their recovery program, they should talk to them about the relapse.

5. *Pick up a white chip.* In AA, a white chip denotes a desire to be abstinent and begin a program of recovery. They should begin again with the first step of Alcoholics Anonymous, "We admitted

we were powerless over alcohol—that our lives had become unmanageable."

6. *Talk with their families and friends.* Although it may be difficult, this is an important step. Families and close friends can provide needed support in starting a new life of recovery.

If adolescents who have relapsed are not willing to take these steps to once again achieve a successful recovery, all is not lost. If drug use continues, however, it may be necessary to institute the procedures discussed earlier—tough love, confrontation, or finally, a court order.

Relapse is not the end of the world. Many consider it to be part of the recovery process. It is, after all, an educational experience. The adolescent can identify the factors that precipitated his relapse, identify his own personal relapse process, and use this information in future relapse prevention efforts.

CONCLUSIONS

Relapse, like recovery, is a process. Several steps lead up to an actual drinking or drug-using episode. A number of factors that lead to relapse have been identified. Relapse is not inevitable. It can be prevented. If relapse does occur, however, the adolescent should take the steps that were given earlier. If the adolescent is not willing to address his ongoing relapse, tough love, confrontation, or court order should be reinstituted. Relapse can be a learning process.

16

Does Drug Abuse Cause Mental Problems?

PRIMARY VERSUS SECONDARY PSYCHIATRIC DISORDERS

Before we can answer the question of whether or not drug abuse causes mental problems, it is first necessary to clarify what we mean by mental problems. The field of psychiatry classifies mental disorders based on signs and symptoms. For instance, a patient with an inability to experience pleasure in things that once gave pleasure, feelings of hopelessness, early morning awakening, and decreased appetite fits the criteria for a psychiatric disorder known as *major depression*.

All substances of abuse affect the brain and change its level of functioning. It should not be surprising then that drugs, as a result of intoxication, overdose, or withdrawal, can produce alterations in mood, ability to reason, and content of thinking. As a result, abuse of various substances can produce signs and symptoms of nearly any psychiatric disorder. However, the signs and symptoms resulting from substance abuse, unlike many true psychiatric disorders, usually abate in a few weeks to months after cessation of drinking or using.

On the other hand, many individuals with true psychiatric disorders also abuse drugs, a condition known as *dual diagnosis*. It can be very difficult, even for trained professionals, to determine if an apparent psychiatric disorder is primary (independent of substance abuse) or secondary (caused by the substance abuse). Common psychiatric conditions that can be mimicked by substance abuse include psychotic disorders, mood disorders, organic brain syndromes, anxiety disorders, and personality disorders.

PSYCHOTIC DISORDERS

Individuals with psychotic disorders have a grossly impaired sense of reality, often coupled with emotional and cognitive disability. They are apt to talk and act bizarrely and have hallucinations such as seeing, hearing, or smelling things that are not there. They may be confused and disoriented. Schizophrenia is the prototype psychotic disorder.

Drug-Induced Psychosis

Hallucinations can occur with intoxication or overdose from the stimulants or hallucinogens and with intoxication from phencyclidine and anabolic steroids; they can also occur as part of the depressant abstinence syndrome. Those hallucinations that occur during alcohol withdrawal may be one of two types. The first occurs as part of *delirium tremens* (DTs) and is always associated with delirium and tremulousness. The second is called *hallucinosis*. In this type, individuals have relatively clear minds and may be aware that their hallucinations are not real.

Cocaine and amphetamine psychosis consist of tactile hallucinations, that is, feeling something crawling on or under the skin ("coke bugs"). Visual and auditory hallucinations may occur, as well as paranoid thinking. Stereotyped behavior, such as compulsive behavior, or picking at the skin, may occur. In its severest form, stimulant psychosis may be indistinguishable from paranoid schizophrenia. For example, one patient spent two years in a state mental institution, incorrectly diagnosed as a paranoid schizophrenic. He was treated with antipsychotic medication the entire time. Two months after discharge he stopped taking the medication on his own and was fine—no psychotic symptoms. It seems that he had been an abuser of amphetamines but denied this to the psychiatrist who admitted him to the hospital. Only a drug screen at the time of admission could have altered the diagnosis.

Phencyclidine psychosis may also be indistinguishable from schizophrenia. Agitation, bizarre behavior, persecutory, grandiose, or somatic delusions, and depersonalization may occur. The comatose state produced by phencyclidine overdose, with open eyes and muscle rigidity, can be confused with catatonic schizophrenia.

Psychosis can occur with high-potency marijuana intoxication and overdose, with depressant intoxication, and with chronic nitrous oxide abuse.

MOOD DISORDERS

Mood disorders are common. The two most severe forms are *bipolar disorder* (manic-depression) and *unipolar disorder* (major depression).

Bipolar Disorder

Episodes of mania in the form of extreme hyperactivity of thought and activity, which are severe enough to interfere with one's ability to function, are necessary for this diagnosis. Most of these individuals also have periods of severe depression.

Unipolar Disorder

Individuals with unipolar disorder have severe bouts of depression, but do not have episodes of mania. A less severe form of chronic depression is known as *dysthymia*.

Drug-Induced Mood Disorders

Depression can be produced by chronic use of depressants, stimulants, and phencyclidines. It may also be a prominent part of alcohol, stimulant, phencyclidine, and anabolic steroid withdrawal. As many as 60 percent of patients entering substance abuse treatment programs are significantly depressed as a result of their drug abuse.

A manic-like state can be produced by stimulant and phencyclidine intoxication or stimulant overdose.

The euphoria and manic-like state produced by anabolic steroids can be confused with bipolar disorder.

ORGANIC BRAIN SYNDROMES

The hallmark of organic brain syndrome is confusion and memory loss. The two most common types are *delirium* and *dementia*.

Delirium

Delirium, which has a multitude of causes, is usually of brief duration, lasting a few hours to a few days. It is a common condition, particularly among people who are physically ill. Individuals with delirium can be confused, act bizarrely, or even become wild. They may appear to be normal or sleepy during the day but deteriorate dramatically at night. Disorientation to time, place, and situation occurs, and memory for recent events is impaired.

Dementia

Dementia results from diffuse organic disease of the cerebral cortex—the thinking and reasoning part of the brain. Dementia has many causes, usually develops slowly, has a long course, and in many cases is irreversible. Early on, individuals undergo subtle changes in personality, impairment of social skills, decrease in range of interests, emotional lability, shallowness of affect, agitation, and gradual loss of intellectual skills. As the condition progresses, they lose memory, undergo changes in mood and personality, lose their orientation, and suffer intellectual impairment, compromised judgment, psychotic symptoms, and language impairment.

The major treatable forms of dementia include the type that results from a series of small strokes, from an obstruction of the outflow tract of cerebrospinal fluid, brain tumors, subdural hematoma (a blood clot on the brain), various infections, miscellaneous disturbances of metabolism, some disorders of major body organs (heart, lungs, kidneys), malnutrition, and ingestion of toxins such as lead, mercury, or pesticides.

The major untreatable forms of dementia are Alzheimer's disease, Parkinson's disease, and Huntington's chorea.

Drug-Induced Organic Brain Syndrome

Delirium can occur with stimulant, phencyclidine, and inhalant intoxication and with overdose of virtually any drug. It can also occur with withdrawal from depressant drugs and opioids.

Dementia most commonly occurs as the result of chronic alcohol abuse, but can occur from chronic inhalant abuse as well. Dementia, in general, may be partly or totally reversible with abstinence, or it may be permanent. The author has seen as patients two adolescent boys who suffered brain damage from gasoline sniffing, resulting in irreversible dementia.

ANXIETY DISORDERS

Anxiety is commonplace. Usually, it is a normal response to stress in a person's life. Anxiety disorders, on the other hand, are fairly uncommon. They involve sufficient distress from anxiety to impair one's ability to function.

Six anxiety disorders are worthy of discussion: (1) adjustment disorder with anxious mood, (2) generalized anxiety disorder, (3) panic disorder, (4) phobic disorder, (5) obsessive–compulsive disorder, and (6) posttraumatic stress disorder.

Adjustment Disorder with Anxious Mood

This disorder is a self-limited response to a significant stress in a person's life, such as a divorce. Mild anxiety, apprehension, and distraction occur. It tends to abate with resolution of the precipitating stress.

Generalized Anxiety Disorder

This disorder consists of more severe and chronic symptoms, including palpitations, diarrhea, cold, clammy extremities, sweating, and urinary frequency. Insomnia, fatigue, sighing, trembling, hypervigilance, and marked apprehension occur. Generalized anxiety disorder by definition lasts longer than six months and in many cases for a lifetime.

Panic Disorder

Panic disorder consists of attacks having dramatic symptoms that last from minutes to hours. They occur in individuals with chronic anxiety and in those without it. Symptoms include heart pounding, chest pain, trembling, choking, sweating, sensation of shortness of breath, disorganization, confusion, and a sense of impending doom or terror. Attacks may come out of the blue or be initiated by crowds or stressful situations. Panic attacks may occur several times daily, weekly, or monthly.

Phobic Disorder

Phobias are fears that are intense, are out of proportion with their stimuli, make little sense even to the sufferers, and lead to an avoidance of the feared objects or situations. When sufficiently distressful or disabling, the condition is termed a *phobic disorder*. Three subtypes of phobic disorder have been identified.

Agoraphobia is a fear of open spaces, crowded spaces, or unfamiliar places. Most individuals with agoraphobia also have panic attacks. Agoraphobia may develop as a result of panic disorder; that is, the unpredictable occurrence of panic attacks causes them to avoid public places for fear of having attacks.

Social phobia is a fear of public speaking, using public lavatories, or eating in public places. Avoidance of these places can be socially crippling.

Simple phobias are fears of things such as thunderstorms, cats, dogs, insects, and mice. Other simple phobias are the fear of closed spaces (claustrophobia) and the fear of heights (acrophobia). The fear of air travel is a common simple phobia.

Obsessive–Compulsive Disorder

Obsessions are repetitive thoughts that are usually unpleasant, always unwanted, and which may be frightening or violent, such as the impulse to leap in front of a car. Individuals may develop compulsions in the form of rituals, such as counting or touching to ward off unwanted happenings or to satisfy an obsession. For example, a person may develop an obsession with dirt, leading to compulsive hand washing rituals. The performing of the ritual serves to reduce the anxiety caused by the obsession.

Posttraumatic Stress Disorder

The characteristic feature of this disorder is the development of symptoms following a psychologically distressful event that is usually outside the range of normal human experience, such as a threat to one's life, to the life of a spouse or child, sudden destruction of one's home, seeing another person killed, or combat or concentration camp experience.

Individuals reexperience the traumatic events in a variety of ways. They may have disturbing thoughts or nightmares about it. Intense psychological stress often occurs when the person is exposed to situations resembling some aspect of the traumatic event or to anniversaries of the event.

Psychic numbing is an integral part of the disorder. The person with posttraumatic stress disorder feels detached from others, is unable to enjoy previously pleasurable activities, and is unable to feel emotions of any kind, especially those associated with intimacy, tenderness, and sexuality. He or she may have trouble falling asleep or staying asleep and have an increased startle response, difficulty concentrating, irritability, and frank aggression.

Drug-Induced Anxiety

Anxiety occurs with chronic alcohol abuse and with stimulant, marijuana, and hallucinogen intoxication and overdose. Anxiety is a prominent feature of depressant and opioid withdrawal.

Panic attacks occur with chronic alcohol use and occur

acutely with stimulant, cannabinoid, and hallucinogen intoxication and with cannabinoid and hallucinogen overdose. They are common in depressant withdrawal. The author knows of one young person who committed suicide by shooting himself because of severe panic attacks resulting from the sudden cessation of use of a sedative drug.

PERSONALITY DISORDERS

The term *personality disorder* refers to personality characteristics of a form of magnitude that is maladaptive, causing poor life functioning. Most personality disorders develop in childhood. They are usually lifelong and resistant to treatment.

Eleven different personality disorders are recognized by the American Psychiatric Association: (1) antisocial, (2) histrionic, (3) borderline, (4) narcissistic, (5) passive–aggressive, (6) paranoid, (7) schizoid, (8) schizotypal, (9) obsessive–compulsive, (10) avoidant, and (11) dependent personality disorders.

Antisocial Personality Disorder

This disorder manifests itself in childhood and adolescence as aggressiveness, fighting, hyperactivity, poor peer relationships, irresponsibility, lying, stealing, truancy, poor school performance, runaway behavior, inappropriate sexual activity, and drug use. In adulthood, criminality, assaultive behavior, self-defeating impulsivity, promiscuity, unreliability, and crippling drug abuse occur. These individuals fail at work, change jobs frequently, receive dishonorable discharges from the service, become abusing parents and neglectful mates, cannot maintain intimate relationships, and spend time in jails and prisons. They are frequently anxious and depressed and tend to make suicide gestures as opposed to serious attempts.

Histrionic Personality Disorder

Individuals with this disorder, when you first get to know them, seem charming, likeable, lively, and seductive. Once you get to know them better you realize that they are emotionally unstable, egocentric, immature, dependent, manipulative, and shallow. They demand attention, are exhibitionistic, and have a limited ability to maintain stable, intimate, interpersonal relationships with either sex. Depression, drug abuse, somatization (physical complaints), and suicide gestures and attempts are common. It is primarily a disorder that occurs in the female sex.

Borderline Personality Disorder

These individuals have complex symptoms, including combinations of anger, anxiety, intense and labile affect, chronic loneliness, boredom, chronic sense of emptiness, volatile interpersonal relationships, identity confusion, and impulsive behavior.

Narcissistic Personality Disorder

These individuals are chronically dissatisfied because of their constant need for admiration and unrealistic expectations. They are impulsive and anxious, have ideas of omnipotence, become quickly dissatisfied with others, and maintain superficial and exploitive interpersonal relationships. When their needs are not met, they become depressed, develop somatic complaints, or display extreme rage.

Passive–Aggressive Personality Disorder

These patients express their hostility passively by intentional inefficiency, negativism, stubbornness, procrastination, and forgetfulness. They are oppositional, resentful, and controlling. As a result, they are irritating and sometimes even infuriating. They suffer anxiety, depression, and have difficulty coping. They have few friends.

Paranoid Personality Disorder

These aloof, emotionally cold people are unjustifiably suspicious, hypersensitive to slights, jealous, and fear intimacy. They tend to be grandiose, rigid, and litigious and, as a result, are isolated and disliked. They accept criticism poorly and blame others for their shortcomings.

Schizoid Personality Disorder

These individuals are seclusive and have little desire or capacity to form interpersonal relationships. They derive little pleasure from social contacts. They can perform well in isolated jobs, such as night watchman. They have a limited emotional range, daydream excessively, and are humorless and aloof.

Schizotypal Personality Disorder

In addition to having features of schizoid personality disorder, these individuals behave peculiarly. They relate strange intrapsychic experiences, reason in odd ways, and are difficult to get to know.

Obsessive–Compulsive Personality Disorder

These individuals, frequently successful men, are inhibited, stubborn, perfectionistic, judgmental, over-conscientious, and rigid. They are chronically anxious, avoid intimacy, and experience little pleasure from life. They are indecisive and demanding and are often perceived as cold and reserved. They are at risk for developing depression and obsessive–compulsive disorder, which has much more pronounced symptoms than the personality form.

Avoidant Personality Disorder

These individuals are shy, lonely, and hypersensitive. Low self-esteem is the hallmark of this disorder. They would rather avoid personal contact than risk any potential social disapproval, even though they are desperate for interpersonal involvement. They suffer from anxiety and depression.

Dependent Personality Disorder

These individuals are excessively passive, unsure, and isolated. They are abnormally dependent on others. This disorder is more common in women and is likely to lead to anxiety and depression, particularly if dependent relationships are threatened.

Drug-Induced Personality Disturbances

Derangement of personality occurs with chronic abuse of all drugs, including alcohol. Addictive behaviors (lying, stealing, cheating) that develop because of substance abuse can be confused with sociopathic personality disorder. Suspiciousness or frank paranoia that results from the abuse of alcohol, stimulants, cannabinoids, hallucinogens, phencyclidine, anabolic steroids, and overdose with stimulants and hallucinogens can be confused with paranoid personality disorder. Isolating, a common symptom of drug addiction, can be confused with schizoid personality disorder, and the low self-esteem of drug-addicted individuals can be mistaken for avoidant personality disorder.

HOW TO MAKE THE DISTINCTION

It is important to distinguish between primary and secondary psychiatric disorders because the overall course of the illness is best predicted by the primary disorder. Primary alcoholism, for instance, has a much better prognosis than antisocial personality disorder.

If the psychiatric signs and symptoms clear with cessation of drug use, it is a safe bet that substance abuse is the primary disorder. On the other hand, if the psychiatric signs and symptoms preceded the onset of substance abuse, existed during an extended period of abstinence, or fail to clear within weeks to months of cessation of drug use, the psychiatric disorder is almost certainly the primary disorder.

Individuals with primary psychiatric disorders may require medication to control their psychiatric symptoms before their substance abuse can be addressed.

CONCLUSIONS

Abuse of alcohol and other drugs can produce symptoms of virtually any psychiatric disorder by virtue of intoxication, overdose, or withdrawal.

Many individuals with true psychiatric disorders also abuse alcohol or other drugs, a condition known as a dual diagnosis. The overall course of the illness is best predicted by the primary disorder; that is, the one that appeared first. Primary psychiatric disorders may have to be treated with medications before the substance abuse problem can be addressed.

Psychiatric symptoms produced by substance abuse are self-limited, abating in a matter of days to weeks after cessation of substance abuse.

Although substance abuse can produce symptoms that are easily confused with those of true psychiatric disorders, it does not cause psychiatric disorders. Substance abuse can, however, trigger mental illness when the illness is in remission. Drug abuse complicates the mental illness by making the symptoms of the illness much worse.

How Are Drugs of Abuse and AIDS Related?

HISTORY OF AIDS

In the summer of 1981, a group of physicians in Los Angeles reported 15 cases of a rare kind of pneumonia in young homosexual men. At about the same time, physicians in New York, San Francisco, and Los Angeles reported 26 cases of an unusual form of skin cancer, again in homosexual young men. Both of these disorders, prior to this, had been seen only in people with severely compromised immune systems. In 1982, the Center for Disease Control (CDC) in Atlanta recognized these as symptoms of a new disease and named it *Acquired Immune Deficiency Syndrome* (AIDS). The virus that causes AIDS was identified in 1983 and is now named *Human Immunodeficiency Virus* (HIV).

PREVALENCE OF AIDS

AIDS has now been reported in all 50 states and in at least 100 countries worldwide. In 1993, the number of cases of AIDS reported in the United States has risen to about 325,000. Overall, HIV is responsible for 19 percent of deaths in young men, and 6 percent of deaths in young women. In addition, it has been estimated that between 1 to 2 million people have been infected with HIV. Most of them are without symptoms and do not know they are infected. They can, of course, pass the virus on to others.

The distribution of AIDS between men and women differs considerably. In the United States, 93 percent of the cases are in men and only 7 percent in women. The difference is due to the fact that the original cases in the United States occurred in homosexual men, and rapidly spread throughout the homosexual community. It is just now beginning a significant spread among heterosexual men and women. In other countries, the disparity of the disease between men and women is not nearly so great.

In 1991 the breakdown of AIDS by group was

Homosexual and bisexual men	71.9%
Intravenous drug users	17.4%
Haitians	4.1%
Persons who have received blood transfusions (hemophiliacs, etc.)	2.0%
Infants born to high risk mothers	1.4%
Heterosexual partners of people with AIDS	1.0%
Others	2.2%

Because 8 percent of cases of AIDS are in bisexual and homosexual men who also have a history of intravenous drug use, one out of four AIDS cases—25.4 percent—involves intravenous drug use.

HIV INFECTION

The Virus

Human immunodeficiency virus has a long latency period. Individuals usually develop symptoms within 4 to 57 months after being infected. Some, however, may not become symptomatic for up to 10 years. The virus is capable of causing severe depression of the immune system, leading to widespread diseases that otherwise do not normally occur.

The virus works by attacking special white blood cells called T4 lymphocytes. The T4 lymphocytes are responsible for activating the system that produces antibodies to fight infection. The virus incorporates itself into the genetic material of the cells (DNA) and codes the DNA to produce large numbers of the virus. Eventually the lymphocytes die so that the white blood cell count drops.

Human immunodeficiency virus can be isolated in high concentrations from the blood and semen of infected people, and to a lesser extent from breast milk, urine, and vaginal secretions. The virus can also be detected in saliva and tears, but in much lower concentrations.

Fortunately, HIV is readily destroyed by drying, heat, ultraviolet light, and common detergents and cleaners such as hand soap, household bleach, and alcohol. Because it is so easily killed, it is not casually transmitted by nonsexual or nonblood-borne routes, such as shaking hands, touching, kissing, or sitting on a toilet seat previously occupied by someone with the infection.

Routes of Infection

Most cases of HIV infection have occurred through four routes: (1) The most common mode of transmission is sexual contact. The risk of infection during intercourse is much higher for women than men. The risk of infection is especially high with anal intercourse, the primary route of infection in homosexual men. (2) Transmission by intravenous drug use occurs through contaminated needles. (3) Infected blood and blood products, during transfusions, can also transmit the virus. (4) Transmission occurs from infected, pregnant women to their unborn children.

Forms of HIV Infection

Individuals infected with HIV may have no signs and symptoms of illness. This is known as the *carrier state*. They may have minimal symptoms, such as swollen lymph nodes, a low-grade fever, nightsweats, and anemia, a condition known as AIDS-related complex (ARC). Finally, they acquire the full-blown disease—AIDS. Acquired immune deficiency syndrome is characterized by all of the signs and symptoms of ARC plus one of several unusual illnesses, such as pneumocystis pneumonia or a form of skin cancer known as Kaposi's sarcoma, which occur only in individuals with severely compromised immune systems. Individuals with the carrier state, ARC, and AIDS are all capable of transmitting the virus to others.

AIDS TESTING

The body's immune system produces antibodies when infected with HIV. The laboratory tests available today detect these antibodies, not the virus itself. Two tests are available for this: the ELISA test and the Western blot test.

The ELISA Test

The *enzyme-linked immunosorbent assay* (ELISA) test is an inexpensive screening test for detection of HIV antibodies in the blood. To perform the test, a laboratory technician adds serum from the blood of the individual being tested to a standard laboratory strain of HIV. If HIV antibodies are present in the person's serum, it interacts with the laboratory HIV to change the color of the solution—a positive test. If HIV antibodies are not present, the solution remains clear—a negative test.

It usually takes about two months for the body to develop antibodies when it is infected with HIV; however, it may take up to 8 months or longer. Tests done after infection occurs but before antibodies are produced give false-negative results.

Because the ELISA test is a screening test, false-positive results do occur; that is, the test can give a positive result when no HIV antibody is actually present in the patient's blood. For this reason, a second, more specific test, the Western blot test, is always performed following positive ELISA tests.

The Western Blot Test

The Western blot test is considerably more expensive than the ELISA test. For this reason, the ELISA test is done first. False-positive results are extremely rare with the Western blot test.

PREVENTION OF AIDS

Since 90.3 percent of HIV infection occurs because of sexual activity or intravenous drug abuse, preventative measures in these areas are extremely important.

Sexual activity. The safest sex is abstinence; however, in this day and time it is unrealistic to believe that all adolescents will abstain from sex to prevent contracting the AIDS virus. This is especially true of drug-abusing adolescents since they tend to be sexually promiscuous. If adolescents are going to have sex, they should limit their number of sex partners. The more partners they have, the greater the risk of contracting HIV.

A condom by itself gives less protection than abstinence, but is safer sex than no protection at all. Diaphragms and birth control pills, of course, give no protection against the AIDS virus.

Intravenous drug use. Fortunately, few adolescents inject drugs intravenously. If needles are used, however, they should not be shared. If shared, they should be sterilized before each use with alcohol or diluted household bleach and rinsed with clean water.

CONCLUSIONS

Although AIDS is primarily a homosexual disease in the United States, it is more a heterosexual disease worldwide. Transmission from person to person occurs primarily by four routes: sexual contact, intravenous drug use with contaminated needles, infected blood and blood products, and transmission from pregnant women to their unborn children. Most infections with the AIDS virus are preventable. There is no cure.

Do I Have Problems of My Own Which I Need to Work On?

GROWING UP IN A DYSFUNCTIONAL FAMILY

It has been my experience that many drug-abusing adolescents come from dysfunctional families. Although there are many causes of dysfunction, a common one is for a parent, or both parents, to have grown up in a dysfunctional family themselves.

Alcoholism is a leading cause of family dysfunction. As alcoholics gradually lose control over their own lives and behavior, they wield more and more power over those close to them. Although they are increasingly dependent on family members for emotional and social support, they play dictator to get it. They control what family members say, what they do, and even what they think. Did you grow up in an alcoholic home? If so, you may need to understand and resolve your own problems before you can tackle your adolescent's problems.

RULES IN THE ALCOHOLIC FAMILY

Because of the tremendous toll alcoholism exacts on a family and its individual members, the family develops a denial system and specific rules to help members cope. In addition, family members tend to assume specific roles.

The person in the family who holds the power makes the rules. In the case of a family with an alcoholic member, that member is the constant focus of every other member's attention and thereby controls what goes on in the family. Thus, the most powerful person in terms of rule making also tends to be the most dysfunctional. The rules are never openly stated, but everyone in the family understands them and lives by them. Sharon Wegscheider-Cruse has identified six such rules:

Rule 1. An alcoholic's use of alcohol is the most important thing in a family's life. The alcoholic is obsessed with maintaining a supply of alcohol. The family is obsessed with cutting it off. The family plans its day around the alcoholic's drinking hours. The alcoholic's drinking is what everything else revolves around.

Rule 2. Someone or something else caused the alcoholic dependency. The increasing tendency for the alcoholic to blame someone or something else for his problems evolves into a rule that gradually becomes imposed on the rest of the family.

Rule 3. The status quo must be maintained at all costs. Alcoholics are afraid to quit drinking, for without alcohol they fear they cannot survive. So, as the rule makers, they make sure that the family remains rigid enough to protect them from change.

Rule 4. Everyone in the family must be an enabler. Family members say they would do anything to get the alcoholic to quit drinking. But at the same time they help, or enable, that person to keep drinking. They make up alibis for the alcoholic, cover up, take over his responsibilities, and accept his rules. They defend these actions on the basis of love, loyalty, or family honor, but the actions only serve to protect the dysfunctional status quo.

Rule 5. No one may discuss what is really going on in the family, either with one another or with outsiders. Feeling threatened, the alcoholic tries to avoid letting people on the outside know about family affairs. The alcoholic also exerts his power to avoid letting family members obtain information and advice from others that might undermine their willingness to enable.

Rule 6. No one may say what he or she is really feeling. The alcoholic is in so much emotional pain that he cannot handle the family's own painful feelings. Therefore, the alcoholic requires everyone to hide his or her feelings. As a result, communication among family members is extremely hampered.

ROLES IN THE ALCOHOLIC FAMILY

Wegscheider-Cruse has identified five roles dysfunctional family members tend to assume in attempts to adapt to the stresses in their lives: (1) the *chief enabler*, (2) the *hero*, (3) the *scapegoat*, (4) the *lost child*, and (5) the *mascot*. Alcoholism is a common cause of dysfunction.

Each role grows out of its own kind of pain, has its own symptoms, offers its own payoffs, and exacts its own price. The oldest child usually becomes the hero, the second child the scapegoat, the next child the lost child, and the youngest the mascot.

Roles tend to change over time, especially as children grow older and leave home. When there are fewer than four children in the family, each child may take on parts of more than one role. Pain and confusion may be particularly overwhelming for an only child.

Since alcoholism is more common in men, we will, for the sake of discussion, consider the alcoholic to be the husband and the chief enabler to be the spouse.

Chief enabler. The spouse usually undertakes the role of chief enabler. She suffers depression, anxiety, and various physical symptoms. The chief enabler feels compelled to try, at all costs, to decrease the chaos that living with an alcoholic produces. In doing so, however, she only helps perpetuate the addiction. Without the chief enabler it would be difficult for the alcoholic to continue drinking. In the early years, she tries to control his drinking by cutting off his supply of alcohol, searching the house for hidden bottles, pouring liquor down the drain, and diluting his drinks. The chief enabler becomes irritated at friends who drink and thereby tempt the alcoholic and stops accepting invitations to parties where alcohol is served. Despite such efforts, the alcoholic continues to drink.

The chief enabler picks up the responsibilities that the alcoholic gives up or simply takes responsibilities away from him. Chief enablers pay bills, fix the plumbing, and discipline the children. They lie to the alcoholic's boss about his absence from work, bail him out of jail, take his side in drunk driving accidents, and drive him to work when he loses his license. The chief enabler continually tries to rescue the alcoholic and will not let him suffer the consequences of his addiction. She makes excuses to the children about his behavior and thus takes the heat off him. This only adds to the children's confusion.

The good intentions of the chief enabler create for the alcoholic an increasingly comfortable environment for the alcoholic to keep on drinking. The alcoholic's meals are cooked, his laundry is done, and his transportation is provided. And just when the chief enabler has had enough, the alcoholic sobers up temporarily, only to begin drinking again at some time in the future. These periods of abstinence keep the chief enabler hanging on for years, hoping that sooner or later she will find the solution to his drinking problem.

The primary feeling the chief enabler develops is anger, although she often masks it with a veneer of concern and unselfishness. She may also feel helpless. She primarily worries and overprotects the alcoholic, her principle defense mechanism being avoidance of crises. Her payoff is temporary peace at any cost and increased self-esteem for doing the "right thing." The price she pays is self-deception and perpetuation of the addiction.

Hero. The hero is the child who feels somehow responsible for the alcoholic's drinking. This responsible, adultlike child takes on the duties of a missing or overburdened parent—preparing meals, worrying about finances, looking out for the welfare of younger brothers or sisters, and trying to keep the family functioning as normally as possible. At school, the hero makes better than average grades, runs for class office, or is an athlete, always working hard to accomplish difficult goals and win the approval of teachers and authority figures.

The hero's characteristic behavior is overachievement. By achieving, the hero believes that maybe the alcoholic parent can be made to feel better and stop drinking. The defense mechanism the hero most often uses is obsessive–compulsive behavior. The hero bases his or her self-worth on performance, and by excelling shows the world that all is right with the family. The hero's payoff is positive attention and praise, resulting in temporary boosts to self-worth. The price the hero pays is eventual workaholism and possible burnout. A hero often grows up to marry an alcoholic or goes into one of the helping professions, such as medicine.

Scapegoat. The scapegoat is the child in the family who feels inferior, often like a victim. For this person, attention for being bad is better than no attention at all. Delinquent and rebellious behavior is common in a scapegoat, behavior that may progress to criminal activity. A scapegoat's defense against emotional pain is substitution—substituting anything for relief of emotional pain. For example, a scapegoat may withdraw from the family and totally substitute peers as a source of approval.

A scapegoat may drop out of school and is an easy prey for cults, the wrong crowd, the latest fad in dress or music, or drug addiction itself. He or she clamors incessantly for attention and a sense of belonging, commonly using anger to cover up fear, sadness, or hurt. The payoff for the person is attention, even if it is negative. The price he or she ultimately pays is rejection and alienation from normal living.

Lost child. This child withdraws from the family in a quiet way, not in the openly defiant way of the scapegoat. The lost child is an adaptor, accepting with a shrug the arbitrarily canceled vacation, the sudden fight, or the unexpected slap. The lost child often separates himself or herself from the rest of the family and spends a great deal of time in his or her room, creating a fantasy world. The lost child is often seen by outsiders as a model child.

The lost child most commonly feels lonely and uses emotional withdrawal and physical retreat as a defense against the painful events occurring in the home. The lost child's payoff is escape from chaos in the family, and the price he pays is social isolation. The lost child is at high risk for suicide.

Mascot. The mascot is the family clown or joker, the one who feels that the chaos at home will suddenly reach a boiling point and explode. The mascot uses humor as a diversion to cheer up the depressing atmosphere and relieve tension. He or she tries to smooth over conflicts before they develop and attempts to heal the hurts of others by giving of himself. The main defense the mascot uses is laughter, tending to laugh or smile when dealing with painful emotions. The mascot's payoff is relief of fear, and the price he or she pays is often psychological emotional immaturity in adulthood.

ADULT CHILDREN OF ALCOHOLICS (ACOAs)

Consequences of Growing Up in a Dysfunctional Family

Having grown up in dysfunctional families, it is no wonder that some of us are far from perfect spouses or parents. The tremendous emotional scars inflicted upon us as children may have led directly to marital discord, emotional depression, vocational instability, and job dissatisfaction. Growing up in an alcoholic home increases the likelihood of growing up to be an alcoholic, marrying an alcoholic, or both, thereby perpetuating the cycle.

Dysfunctional Characteristics of ACOAs

Children growing up in dysfunctional families tend to carry into adult life certain dysfunctional characteristics that affect their ability to parent effectively. Janet Woititz has identified twelve characteristics of ACOAs. Do any of them apply to you?

1. *Adult children of alcoholics guess what normal is.* Adult children of alcoholics grew up in homes that were not "normal" as a result of alcoholism. They simply have no experience with what is normal. They often bring a fantasized concept of the perfect family into a marriage, thus making life very difficult and unrealistic.

2. *Adult children of alcoholics have trouble following a project through from beginning to end.* In the typical alcoholic family there are a lot of promises. The great job was always just around the corner, the big deal was almost always about to be made, the work that needed to be done around the house would be done, but these things never happened. Thus, ACOAs had a role model for procrastination. Not only that, they really never had anyone to show them how to carry a project through from beginning to end. As a result, they have difficulty following a project through from beginning to end.

3. *Adult children of alcoholics lie when it would be just as easy to tell the truth.* Lying is basic to the alcoholic family. The first and most basic lie is the family's denial of the problem. The pretense that everything at home is in order is a lie. The nonalcoholic parent lies to cover up for the alcoholic and makes excuses for him not fulfilling obligations, not being on time, or not showing up when expected. Alcoholics make a lot of promises that turn out to be lies. Lying tends to become a habit in the alcoholic's household. It's not surprising that the children carry this habit over into adulthood.

4. *Adult children of alcoholics judge themselves without mercy.* As a child, ACOAs never felt they were good enough. They were constantly criticized. Since they were never able to meet the standards of perfection expected of them in childhood, they carried this feeling into adulthood. Whatever they do is not quite good enough. They have trouble accepting compliments. Their judgment of others is not nearly as harsh as their judgment of themselves.

5. *Adult children of alcoholics have difficulty having fun.* The childhoods of ACOAs were probably not much fun. They seldom heard their parents laughing and joking. Life was a very serious

business. They grew up with the same attitude. They tend not to join in games because they are afraid of looking foolish or making a mistake; that is, not playing the game perfectly. They have difficulty having fun. They take themselves very seriously.

6. *Adult children of alcoholics have difficulty with intimate relationships.* It is difficult for ACOAs to have healthy, intimate relationships. This occurs because they do not have a frame of reference for a healthy, intimate relationship since they did not grow up in one. They grew up in an inconsistent parent–child relationship, loved one day and rejected the next. As a result, they developed a fear of being close, yet still feel the need for intimacy. Furthermore, they have developed a fear of abandonment which causes them to lack confidence in their present relationships.

7. *Adult children of alcoholics overreact to changes over which they have no control.* Growing up, ACOAs were not in charge of their lives. The alcoholic's lifestyle was inflicted on them. As a result, they fear that when a change is made without them participating in it, they will lose control of their lives. Therefore, they tend to overreact. They simply don't adjust to change very well. They are often accused of being controlling, rigid, and lacking in spontaneity.

8. *Adult children of alcoholics constantly seek approval and confirmation.* Children begin to believe who they are from the messages they get from their parents. As they get older, these messages become internalized and contribute significantly to their self-images. As children, these messages were confusing, so they grew up lacking self-confidence. They feel that anyone who would care about them must not be worth very much. They constantly seek approval and confirmation of their self-worth.

9. *Adult children of alcoholics usually feel different from other people.* Adult children of alcoholics assume that in any group of people, everyone else feels comfortable and they are the only ones who feel awkward. They feel different from other people. When growing up, they became isolated. As a result, they did not develop the social skills necessary to feel comfortable as part of a group. It is difficult for ACOAs to believe that they can be accepted

because of who they are and that acceptance does not have to be earned.

10. *Adult children of alcoholics are super responsible or super irresponsible.* Adult children of alcoholics tried unsuccessfully as children to please their parents by doing more and more. Some continued this characteristic into adulthood while others reached the point where they realized it didn't really matter and began doing as little as they could. Those that continued to strive feel that if they are not perfect they will be rejected, so they tend to be super responsible. They subject themselves to enormous pressure trying to be the perfect spouse, the perfect parent, the perfect friend, and the perfect employee. Those who are super irresponsible tend to suffer from procrastination. They have trouble getting started.

11. *Adult children of alcoholics are extremely loyal.* Family members of alcoholics are extremely loyal and hang in long after reason dictates they should leave. No one walks away just because the going gets tough. This sense allows the ACOA to remain in relationships that are better dissolved. Since making a friend or developing a relationship is so difficult, once it is made it tends to be permanent. The fact that they may be treated poorly doesn't matter. It can be rationalized.

12. *Adult children of alcoholics are impulsive.* Adult children of alcoholics grew up in a home in which impulsive behavior by the alcoholic was the norm. No serious consideration was given to what happened the last time nor what the consequences would be this time. The reality in the alcoholic home was that if it were not done immediately, it never got done. Adult children of alcoholics tend to be impulsive, leading to confusion, self-loathing, and loss of control over their environment. They spend an excessive amount of time cleaning up the mess.

SUPPORT GROUPS FOR ACOAs

Because of the needs of ACOAs, much like the need of alcoholics for AA, a support organization for ACOAs evolved which adapted the 12 steps of AA for its own purpose. Two steps, 1 and 12, were modified. Step 1 became, "We admitted we were powerless over *the past*—that our lives had become unmanageable." Step 12 became, "Having had a spiritual awakening as the result of these steps, we tried to carry this message to *others*, and to practice these principles in all our affairs."

Adult children of alcoholics meetings take place weekly and consist of leaderless support groups, much like AA meetings. Members work on, with the help of other members, their dysfunctional characteristics. If you feel like you have ACOA issues, by all means locate and join a support group.

CONCLUSIONS

Many substance-abusing adolescents come from dysfunctional families. Alcoholism is a leading cause of this dysfunction. Families with chemically dependent members tend to develop dysfunctional rules by which they live, and they tend to assume certain dysfunctional roles.

Children growing up in alcoholic families may carry certain dysfunctional characteristics into adult life that can affect their ability to parent effectively. Support groups for these adults have evolved.

IV

Drugs of Abuse

19

Pharmacology of Drugs of Abuse

An understanding of the basic principles of pharmacology is essential to the understanding of how drugs of abuse exert their harmful effects.

PHARMACOKINETICS

Four major processes determine both the intensity and duration of a drug's action: (1) absorption, (2) distribution, (3) metabolism, and (4) excretion. The branch of pharmacology that is concerned with these four processes is called *pharmacokinetics*.

Absorption

Route of Administration

Drugs can be ingested orally, insufflated (snorted up the nose), inhaled, or injected with a needle. Ingested dugs must cross the intestinal wall to reach the bloodstream. Others, such as alcohol, may be partially absorbed in the stomach. Drugs that are insufflated, such as cocaine, must cross the lining of the nose. Drugs whose vapors are inhaled (e.g., amyl nitrate and nitrous oxide), or which are combusted and then inhaled (e.g., nicotine, marijuana, and cocaine), must cross the pulmonary membrane to reach the bloodstream. Many drugs, such as cocaine, methamphetamine, and heroin, can be injected subcutaneously, intramuscularly, or intravenously.

The site of absorption can markedly affect the rapidity of onset, as well as the degree of effect of the drug. Cocaine in the form of chewed coca leaf, for example, is slowly absorbed in the mouth and small intestine; it is absorbed more rapidly and reaches a higher peak when smoked. In fact, smoking cocaine approximates the rapid delivery of intravenous cocaine to the brain because drugs that are inhaled have rapid access to the bloodstream through the pulmonary membrane. Because the blood flow from the heart passes through the capillaries of the lungs, the delivery of a drug from the lungs to the brain is enhanced.

Diffusion

Diffusion of most drugs through biological membranes is passive and depends on both the concentration of the drug and the ability of the drug to pass through the membrane. Drugs move across membranes from areas of higher concentrations to areas of lower concentration by virtue of their kinetic activity. In addition, a drug must have certain chemical properties to pass through membranes easily: relatively small molecule size, adequate solubility in lipids, and lack of electric charge.

Partition Coefficient

Biological membranes behave as if they are lipid solvents. As a result, how well a drug passes through a membrane depends in part on its lipid solubility. The *partition coefficient* is a measure of the relative solubility of a drug. It is defined as the ratio of the concentration of the drug dissolved in oil to its concentration when it is dissolved in water. The higher the partition coefficient the easier the drug passes through a membrane. The cellular barrier of the blood vessel wall, however, has gaps between the cells so that even drugs with low partition coefficients pass with ease.

Effects of pH

The degree of acidity or alkalinity of a solution (pH) markedly alters the degree of charge on drugs that ionize the solution as weak acids or bases. A weak acid will be least charged in an acidic fluid and most charged in an alkaline fluid. On the other hand, a weak base will be most charged in an acidic fluid and least charged in an alkaline fluid. The greater the charge of a drug the less lipid soluble, and the more water soluble, the drug is. The converse is also true. Therefore, a weak acid, such as phenobarbital, in an alkaline solution will tend to be trapped on one side of a membrane because of its charge. A weak base, such as methadone, will be least charged in an alkaline solution and, therefore, tend to be trapped on the acidic side of a membrane, such as in the lumen of the stomach.

In summary, drugs are absorbed through biological membranes by a system of passive movement that is characterized by (1) a tendency to move from higher concentrations to lower concentrations, (2) a tendency for more lipid-soluble drugs to cross membranes more readily, and (3) a tendency for charged particles of weak acids or bases to be trapped on one side of a membrane.

Distribution

The simplest compartments of distribution for drugs can be described in terms of extracellular and intracellular water. *Extra-*

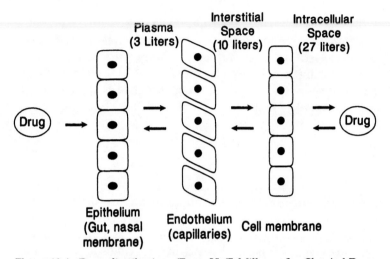

Figure 19.1. Drug distribution. (From H. T. Milhorn, Jr., *Chemical Dependence: Diagnosis, Treatment, and Prevention*, Springer-Verlag, New York, 1990. Reprinted with permission.)

cellular water can further be subdivided into plasma (intravascular) and interstitial (extravascular) fluids (Fig. 19.1). Drugs that stay in the plasma distribute to 3 liters of body fluid. Charged drugs may distribute only through extracellular fluid (3 + 10 = 13 liters) since they cannot readily cross cell membranes. Drugs that are water soluble and cross membranes readily, such as ethanol, may be distributed into all body water (3 + 10 + 27 = 40 liters).

Some drugs in the plasma compartment are in solution while others are combined with plasma proteins, most commonly albumin. A dynamic equilibrium exists between free drug and protein-bound drug. The binding constitutes a reservoir for the drug and may significantly affect the distribution of the drug to other sites in the body. Hence, both the effect of the drug and its rate of elimination may be retarded. Methadone, for instance, has a relatively prolonged effect and a prolonged persistence in the body, in part because of it is highly bound to plasma protein.

Volume of Distribution

The *volume of distribution* (V_d) of a drug is a ratio of the amount of drug in the body divided by the concentration of the drug in the plasma at that time. It is usually calculated by dividing the initial dose (D_0) of drug by an extrapolated concentration at time zero (C_0) as shown in Fig. 19.2. The alpha phase is due to drug distribution. The beta phase is due to metabolism and excretion.

Drug Accumulation in Adipose Tissues

Fatty (adipose) tissue can act as a storage depot for lipid-soluble drugs. Because blood flow through fat is rather slow, drugs that accumulate in fat, such as the major psychoactive component of marijuana (THC), tend to stay there for long periods of time, and are usually released back into the bloodstream slowly after use of the drug has stopped. This can result in positive drug screens for a protracted period of time.

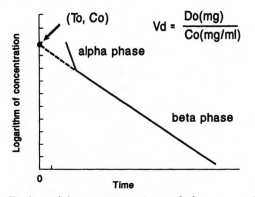

Figure 19.2. Decline of drug concentration and plasma over time. (From H. T. Milhorn, Jr., *Chemical Dependence: Diagnosis, Treatment, and Prevention*, Springer-Verlag, New York, 1990. Reprinted with permission.)

The Blood–Brain Barrier

The capillary endothelial cells of the central nervous system (CNS) greatly reduce the ability of many drug molecules to diffuse across the membrane and reach effective concentrations in the brain. The blood–brain barrier probably evolved to protect the cells of the brain against foreign substances. Only drugs that are very lipid soluble can cross the blood–brain barrier well and produce achievable actions in the brain. Such drugs include anesthetic gases, alcohol, sedatives, and hypnotics.

The Placental Barrier

The capillary network of the placenta limits the ability of some drugs in the maternal circulation to reach the fetal circulation. The placental barrier serves as a means to protect the fetus against potentially harmful drug effects. Nevertheless, many drugs that enter the maternal circulation, including alcohol, nicotine, cocaine, and heroin, can cross the placental barrier, and may cause fetal dependence, toxicity, and/or birth defects.

Metabolism

Most drugs that enter the body are changed by a series of chemical reactions known as *metabolism*, or *biotransformation*. This is one of the two major processes the body has for reducing the amount of active drug in the body. The other is *excretion*. The major site of drug metabolism is the liver.

Metabolites

Biotransformation transforms a drug into one or more other substances called *metabolites*. Metabolites are generally less active pharmacologically and, therefore, less toxic to the body. They are also more water soluble so they can be excreted more readily by the kidneys. Some drugs are totally metabolized into other compounds before they are excreted. Others undergo no metabolism and are excreted unchanged. Most drugs, however, undergo both processes, with most of the drug being metabolized and the rest excreted without prior metabolism.

Hepatic Drug Metabolism

Most liver cells, or *hepatocytes*, contain many complex and active enzyme systems that metabolize drugs. Two of these are the microsomal and the nonmicrosomal enzyme systems. The *microsomal enzymes* are found primarily in the endoplasmic reticulum of the hepatocyte. They metabolize drugs with widely differing structures, such as phenobarbital, amphetamines, and meperidine (Demerol). They perform two basic types of chemical reactions on drugs, synthetic and nonsynthetic. Synthetic reactions involve chemically combining the parent or some of its metabolites with another compound such as an amino acid or a sugar. This is referred to as *conjugation*. Nonsynthetic reactions oxidize (combine with oxygen), reduce, or hydrolyze (combine with water) the parent drug or its metabolites.

The *nonmicrosomal enzyme system* also metabolizes drugs nonspecifically. Alcohol dehydrogenase, the enzyme that metabolizes ethanol, for example, also metabolizes ethylene glycol.

Drugs administered orally pass through the liver, which provides the liver cells with an opportunity to transform drugs that have just entered the body. Many orally administered drugs can be significantly inactivated the first time they pass through the liver so that their concentrations in the blood are considerably less than they would otherwise be. This phenomenon is known as the *first-pass effect*.

Several important factors, however, can alter the liver's ability to metabolize drugs, and therefore can dramatically influence a person's response to the drug. Such factors include the person's age, nutritional status, inherited ability, and presence of liver disease.

Types of Enzymatic Reactions

Two types of enzymatic reactions occur, first order and zero order. In a *first-order reaction*, the concentration of the drug is well below the level that would saturate the binding sites of the enzyme. The drug is, therefore, metabolized at a rate proportional to its concentration. Most drugs undergo first-order kinetics. In a *zero-order reaction*, the binding sites on the enzymes are saturated. The rate of metabolism, therefore, is constant. Ethanol is an important example of a drug that obeys zero-order kinetics. Some drugs, such as phenytoin (Dilantin), obey first-order kinetics at lower concentrations and zero-order kinetics at higher concentrations.

Enzyme Inhibition and Induction

Drug-metabolizing enzymes may be inhibited or induced, meaning stimulated. Inhibition may be competitive or noncompetitive. *Competitive inhibition* occurs when a substance with a structure similar to the correct one combines reversibly with the active sites of the enzyme. This type of inhibition may be overcome by increasing the concentration of the correct substance. One example of competitive inhibition is the inhibition of acetaldehyde dehydrogenase (an enzyme in the metabolism chain of alcohol) by disulfiram (Antabuse). This results in a severe reaction when alcohol is ingested due to the fact that the toxic acetaldehyde formed by the metabolism of the alcohol cannot be broken down to less toxic substances. *Noncompetitive inhibition* occurs when an agent, unrelated in structure to the drug, binds in a distorted manner to prevent normal interaction between the drug and the enzyme. This form of inhibition cannot be overcome by increasing the concentration of the drug.

Microsomal enzymes undergo a quantitative increase in metabolizing ability, known as *induction*, when persistently exposed to a variety of drugs. Since most drugs that do this are lipid soluble, entering the liver cells is apparently necessary for drugs to cause enzyme induction. Phenobarbital is the most commonly known drug to do this. A few drugs, such as meprobamate (Equanil, Miltown) and glutethimide (Doriden), may, by enzyme induction, hasten their own metabolism.

Excretion

Renal Excretion

Drugs, or their metabolites, are excreted primarily in the urine. Three processes affect the fate of a drug once it has reached the kidneys: (1) glomerular filtration, or the portion of the plasma that is filtered through the kidneys, (2) tubular secretion, the secretion of interstitial fluid and its contents into the renal tubules for elimination in the urine, and (3) tubular reabsorption, the portion of the fluid and its contents filtered through the kidneys that is reabsorbed and does not enter the urine. Glomerular filtration and tubular secretion increase the amount of drug eliminated by the body, while tubular reabsorption reduces the amount of drug eliminated. Compounds that are water soluble remain in the urine after glomerular filtration or tubular secretion and are excreted from the body. Those that are lipid soluble may passively diffuse across the renal tubular wall back into the bloodstream (tubular reabsorption), only to repeat the cycle over and over. Without the metabolic conversion of lipid-soluble drugs, such as phenobarbital, to water-soluble metabolites, these drugs would remain in the body for months to years.

By changing the pH of the urine, it is possible to change the degree of charge of some compounds, rendering them less lipid-soluble and, hence, more readily excreted from the body in urine. Alkalinization of the urine by ingestion of an alkaline substance, for example, may enhance the excretion of some weak acids, such as phenobarbital. Similarly, acidification of the urine by ingesting an acid substance may increase the excretion of some weak bases, such as amphetamines, methadone, and phencyclidine (PCP).

Hepatic Excretion

The liver excretes some drugs via the bile into the duodenum. Probably the majority of these compounds are not excreted in significant amounts in the feces but instead are reabsorbed by the intestines to eventually be excreted by the kidneys. Glutethimide is thought to be intensively subjected to this *interhepatic circulation*, thus explaining why the drug persists in the body so long after an overdose.

Other Sites of Excretion

An alternate, but less important route of excretion is the lungs. The characteristic breath odor of the individual who has been drinking alcohol is due to respiratory excretion of the drug. Alcohol concentrations in the breath are so closely related to blood alcohol levels that they are used to determine whether a person has a blood alcohol level above the legal limit for operating a motor vehicle. In addition, varying amounts of some drugs are excreted in feces, sweat, breast milk, and saliva.

Steady-State Relationships

The *half-life* of a drug is defined as the time required for the serum concentration of the drug to fall to 50 percent of its previous level. Only drugs that obey first-order kinetics can be described in terms of half-life. The time for drugs which obey zero-order kinetics, such as alcohol, to fall to 50 percent of their previous level depends on the dose. The greater the dose, the longer the amount of time required for this to occur. The half-life of a drug is determined by the interaction between absorption, distribution, metabolism, and excretion.

When a drug is administered at intervals less than, or equal to, the half-life of the drug, it will begin to accumulate in the blood because some of the previous dose is still present with each additional dose. Eventually a point of balance—steady-state—is reached in which the rate of excretion and metabolism is equal to the rate of administration. The dose markedly affects the steady-state level but does not affect the time required to reach it. The time reported to reach a steady state is a function only of the half-life of the drug. The steady-state concentration, whatever it is going to be, will be reached in 4 or 5 half-lives of the drug, regardless of dose size.

PHARMACODYNAMICS

The study of how drugs exert their effects is called *pharmacodynamics*. It focuses on how the molecules of most drugs interact with specific receptors on target cells, how a biological response occurs, the relationship of the dose and the resultant response to a drug, and the way one drug can alter the response to another one.

Receptors

Many drugs produce their effects by interacting with specific macromolecules that are usually located on a cell's outer membrane. These specific interaction sites are called *receptors*. The shape, size, electrical charge, and other properties of the receptor surface are compatible with those of the specific drug molecules that interact with it. This interaction is often described with a lock and key analogy (Fig. 19.3). *Agonists* interact with the receptor to form a drug–receptor complex, and in doing so alter cell function to cause a response. Agonists whose characteristics exactly match those of the receptor cause a strong response (Fig. 19.3A), while agonists that do not precisely match the receptor cause a weaker response (Figs. 19.3B and C). Some drugs, called *antagonists*, have properties that allow them to bind to a receptor but produce no response at all (Fig. 19.3D). By binding to the receptors, they prevent the formation of an agonist–receptor complex and thereby block the response that would ordinarily occur. Naloxone (Narcan)

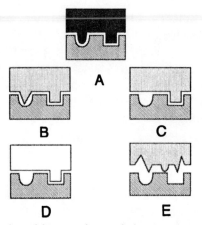

Figure 19.3. Lock-and-key analogy of drug receptor interaction. (A) Strong agonist, (B) and (C) weak agonist, (D) antagonist, and (E) no interaction. (From H. T. Milhorn, Jr., *Chemical Dependence: Diagnosis, Treatment, and Prevention*, Springer-Verlag, New York, 1990. Reprinted with permission.)

and naltrexone (Trexan) are examples of opioid antagonists. They will actually displace drugs such as morphine and hydromorphone (Dilaudid) from the receptors. Some analgesic drugs, such as pentazocine (Talwin) and nalbuphine (Nubain), have varying degrees of both agonist and antagonist activity. They will precipitate withdrawal symptoms in narcotic addicts. Finally, drugs that do not match receptor sites will not interact at all (Fig. 19.3E).

The binding of a drug molecule to its receptor is the first step leading to a response; in many cases this activates a second step. Drugs that cause muscle contraction, for example, do so by first forming a drug–receptor complex on the muscle cell. This activates adenyl cyclase, an enzyme that increases the formation of cyclic adenosine monophosphate (cAMP). In turn, cAMP increases the flow of calcium ions into the cell, activating the contractile proteins and causing muscle contraction.

Dose-Response Curves

Dose-Response Plots

Discussion of drug–receptor interaction is usually done using semilogarithmic dose-response plots of drug plasma concentration versus physiological response (Fig. 19.4). The semilogarithmic plot has several advantages: a wide range of doses can be displayed, and the curves are usually S-shaped with a linear middle segment, which implies that binding to the receptors is a first-order process within this linearity, that is, the amount of drug binding to the receptors is directly proportional to the drug's concentration. Drugs producing the same effects by the same mechanism produce dose-response curves whose linear segments parallel each other. When two drugs act individually by binding to the same receptors, they produce the same maximum response, called a *plateau*. The plateau means that all receptors have become

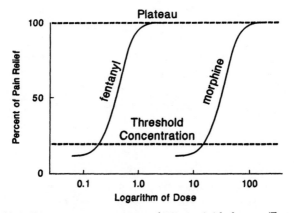

Figure 19.4. Dose-response curves of two opioid drugs. (From H. T. Milhorn, Jr., *Chemical Dependence: Diagnosis, Treatment, and Prevention*, Springer-Verlag, New York, 1990. Reprinted with permission.)

saturated. In addition, there is a minimum plasma concentration of a drug that is necessary to initiate a response. The amount of drug that produces this minimum concentration is called the *threshold dose*.

Affinity, Potency, and Efficacy

The tendency of a drug to be bound at given receptor sites is known as its *affinity*. In Fig. 19.4, fentanyl produces a response at a lower dose than morphine. Fentanyl, therefore, has a greater affinity for the receptors, and is said to be more potent. *Potency* indicates the dose of a drug needed to produce a given response when compared to the dose of another drug required to produce the same response. Fentanyl and morphine reach the same plateau. Therefore, they have the same *efficacy* (response-producing ability) despite differing potencies. Drugs that plateau at lower maximum responses than other drugs are said to be less efficacious.

Synaptic Transmission

Transmission of a nerve signal from one neuron to the next in the brain requires the action of a chemical substance called a *neurotransmitter*. Drugs of abuse produce their effects by altering the function of these substances at neural synapses.

Synaptic Function

Action potentials move down the *presynaptic neuron* and reach the nerve terminal where they cause release of calcium ions. These, in turn, act on *storage vesicles* to initiate the release of neurotransmitter molecules. The neurotransmitter molecules then cross the *synaptic cleft* where they momentarily interact with receptors on the *postsynaptic neuron*. Activation of the receptors causes the conversion of adenyl cyclase to cAMP which, in turn, initiates action potentials in the postsynaptic neuron. After the brief interaction with the *postsynaptic receptors*, the neurotransmitter molecules tend to return to the presynaptic vesicles for storage and reuse. A portion of the neurotransmitter molecules is rendered inactive by a specific enzyme in the synaptic cleft. Synaptic transmission is very rapid, requiring only about 1/1000 of one second.

Effects of Drugs on Synaptic Function

As we discussed earlier, drugs alter synaptic function by a variety of mechanisms: (1) administration of neurotransmitter precursors may increase the availability of a neurotransmitter in the presynaptic vesicles, (2) some drugs decrease the activity of the metabolizing enzyme in the synaptic cleft, making more of the neurotransmitter available at the postsynaptic receptors, (3) antagonistic drugs may displace neurotransmitter molecules from the postsynaptic receptors, (4) a drug may mimic the activity of the neurotransmitter to increase receptor activity, (5) a drug may block access to the receptor, (6) a drug may block reuptake of neurotransmitter molecules from the synaptic cleft; in doing so, it increases neurotransmitter availability at the postsynaptic receptors, and (7) a drug may facilitate release of neurotransmitter molecules from the presynaptic vesicles.

Upregulation and Downregulation

Upregulation and downregulation involve the development of increased or decreased numbers of postsynaptic receptors, respectively. As an example of *upregulation*, consider the following: some psychotic patients require antipsychotic medications, such as chlorpromazine, for years, producing a prolonged dopamine receptor blockade. This may cause the development of additional postsynaptic receptors in an attempt to return synaptic transmission toward normal. If removal of the neuroleptic blockage occurs, the patient may develop tardive dyskinesia, a movement disorder, due to activation of the excess receptors by normal amounts of dopamine. When an excessive degree of activation of postsynaptic receptors occurs over time, such as with heroin dependence, a decrease in the number of receptors occurs in an attempt to return synaptic transmission toward normal. This phenomenon is known as *downregulation*.

Neurotransmitters Affected by Psychoactive Substances

Six neurotransmitters [gamma-aminobutyric acid (GABA), acetylcholine, norepinephrine, dopamine, serotonin, and beta-endorphin] account for most of the symptoms seen with the most commonly abused drugs in the United States.

Kindling

If a drug is capable of producing some symptom, regular use of the drug at the original dose level may evoke the symptom, not after the first dose, but after multiple doses, a phenomenon known as *kindling*. The paranoid schizophreniform reaction to cocaine is an example of kindling. It may not occur with the first dose, the second dose, or even the third dose, but develops after multiple doses over a period of time.

TOLERANCE AND CROSS TOLERANCE

Most, if not all, psychoactive drugs lose some effect with repeated use. The individual who wishes to achieve a specific effect, such as becoming "high," must use larger and larger doses, a phenomenon known as *tolerance*. Tolerance is traditionally divided into dispositional and pharmacodynamic tolerance. *Dispositional tolerance* involves an increased rate of metabolism, almost always because of hepatic microenzyme induction. This probably plays a small role in the development of tolerance to drugs of abuse. The major cause of tolerance, *pharmacodynamic tolerance*, takes place at the cellular level in the brain, perhaps resulting in part from neurotransmitter downregulation. Dependent individuals simply function better at a given serum level of a drug than the nontolerant individual. The author has seen a number of alcoholics with blood alcohol levels greater than 0.4 gm/100 ml who were still walking and talking. Most nontolerant individuals would be approaching a comatose state at this level.

Tolerance is not an all-or-none phenomenon; it develops to some aspects of drug actions but not to others. Amphetamine abusers, for example, may develop tolerance to the cardiovascular and euphoric effects of the drug, but remain at high risk for the psychosis-producing effect.

Cross tolerance is the development of tolerance to drugs in the same class as the abused drug. This occurs without actual use of the drugs. The heroin addict, for example, will automatically develop tolerance to other opioid drugs, such as morphine, hydromorphone, or codeine, as he becomes tolerant to the effects of the heroin. The heroin addict who is injured, for example, will not respond to the usual dose of narcotic medication for pain. Cross tolerance develops in alcoholics to other central nervous system depressant drugs, such as barbiturates, benzodiazepines, meprobamate, and gaseous anesthetics. Cross tolerance can occur among members of other drug groups as well.

PHYSICAL DEPENDENCE
AND ABSTINENCE SYNDROME

The term *physical dependence* is used to distinguish those drugs that, upon cessation of use, are associated with an *abstinence syndrome*; that is, the occurrence of withdrawal symptoms. The most dramatic abstinence syndrome is produced by drugs that depress the central nervous system, such as alcohol, barbiturates, and benzodiazepines. It results from central nervous system hyperactivity that produces tachycardia, hypertension, anxiety, insomnia, and, sometimes, seizures. Death does occasionally occur, particularly when the abstinence syndrome takes place in the absence of medical supervision. Cessation of use of other drugs, such as cocaine, amphetamines, and phencyclidine, produces much less dramatic withdrawal symptoms. In fact, for many years cocaine was thought not to produce physical dependence because its rather mild abstinence syndrome was not recognized. The opioid drugs, such as heroin and morphine, produce an intermediate abstinence syndrome. Central nervous system hyperactivity occurs but not to the extent produced by the CNS depressant group of drugs; it is not life threatening to the user. Some drugs, such as LSD and mescaline, are not associated with an abstinence syndrome.

SET AND SETTING

Other factors that have an impact on the effects of a drug are *set* and *setting*.

Set

Set refers to the physiological and psychological state of the user.

Physiological Set

General physical health, body size, condition of the liver and kidneys, the amount of food in the stomach, other drugs in the body, and how well rested the body is are some of the variables that comprise one's physiological set. For example, drinking alcohol on an empty stomach leads to more rapid absorption and, consequently, more rapid intoxication.

Psychological Set

The expectation of the user, based on his previous experiences, stories he has heard, and what he has seen with other drug users, is the most important aspect of psychological set. Mood, attitude, and general personality characteristics also contribute to psychological set. These factors account for the well-known placebo effects of drugs.

Setting

Setting refers to the environment in which a drug is used. A novice user might experience a somewhat different effect when using a drug at a party where loud rock music is being played as opposed to using it at home alone.

CONCLUSIONS

The branch of pharmacology concerned with absorption, distribution, metabolism, and excretion of drugs is known as pharmacokinetics. The study of how drugs exert their effects on the body is known as pharmacodynamics.

Drugs produce their effects by altering the ability of nerve signals to cross a gap, known as a synapse, between two nerve cells. They do so by affecting the effectiveness of chemical substances known as neurotransmitters.

The effect a drug has on an individual is also determined by the physiological and psychological state (set) and the environment (setting).

20

Alcohol

Some 350,000 8th-grade children are binge drinkers; this number climbs to 690,000 for 10th graders. Problems caused by young people abusing alcohol include bad grades, school dropouts, accidents, assaults, rapes, and death.

About one-third of youths who have committed serious crimes consumed alcohol just prior to the offense. Many teenage suicides involved frequent use of alcohol or other drugs. Alcohol is a factor in more than one-half of all rapes among college students. Nearly 40 percent of drownings and 75 percent of fatal accidents with all-terrain vehicles involve the use of alcohol.

THE ALCOHOL DRUGS

Alcohol (ethanol) is usually abused in the forms of beer, wine, and liquor or whiskey. Wine coolers, which contain about the same amount of alcohol as beer, have become popular drinks of adolescents. At around 5 percent, beer has the lowest alcohol content. Wines range from 9 to 12.5 percent, and liquors and whiskeys are the highest at 40 to 50 percent. A 12-ounce can of beer contains about the same amount of alcohol as a 5-ounce glass of wine and a shot (1.5 ounces) of liquor or whiskey; all are equally addicting. *Proof* equals twice the concentration; for example, 80 proof whiskey contains 40 percent alcohol by volume.

HISTORY

Alcoholic beverages have been used by man since the dawn of history. Breweries can be traced back 6000 years to ancient Egypt and Babylonia. The oldest alcoholic drinks—beers and wines—were produced by fermentation and as a result had relatively low alcohol contents. Distillation, a process to increase the alcohol content, was introduced to Europe in the middle ages by the Arabs. Alcohol was believed to be a remedy for practically all illnesses. The word *whiskey* comes from Gaelic, meaning "water of life."

Early colonists commonly drank beer and wine with meals, but did not tolerate drunkenness; however, after the year 1725, people increasingly drank alcoholic beverages of higher alcohol content, and excess drinking became not only tolerated, but admired—it was immoral, but it was manly. In 1789, a movement began that opposed widespread intemperance, and which later promoted abstinence. It culminated, in 1920, in the passage of the Eighteenth Amendment of the U.S. Constitution, which prohibited the manufacture, transportation, or sale of intoxicating beverages except for medical or sacramental purposes. "Intoxicating beverage" was later redefined to allow the sale and consumption of beer with 3.2 percent alcohol content. Unfortunately, prohibition simply did not work, and in 1934 the Twenty-first Amendment replaced the Eighteenth, ending prohibition.

In 1935, a surgeon named Dr. Bob Smith and a stockbroker named Bill Wilson, two hopeless alcoholics, discovered that they could stay sober by helping each other, and thus founded Alcoholics Anonymous. In 1939, they wrote the "Big Book" of Alcoholics Anonymous. In 1945, Mrs. Marty Mann founded the National Council on Alcoholism (NCA), a volunteer group dedicated to eradicating the stigma of alcoholism and educating the general public about its treatment and prevention. The World Health Organization (WHO) acknowledged alcoholism as an illness in 1951, and in 1956 the American Medical Association (AMA) declared alcoholism to be a disease. E. M. Jellinek published his landmark book, *The Disease Concept of Alcoholism*, in 1960, and the American Psychiatric Association recognized alcoholism as a disease in 1965.

In 1970, the Hughes Act established the National Institute of Alcohol Abuse and Alcoholism (NIAAA) at the federal level. The Hughes Act authorized financial assistance to states, communities, organizations, institutions, and individuals; funded research, education, training, and treatment and rehabilitation programs; and withdrew federal funds from hospitals that refused to treat alcoholics.

ACTIONS

The specific effects of alcohol on the brain depend on the blood alcohol level (BAL). In the nontolerant individual, effects related to specific BALs are:

BAL (gm/100 ml)	Effects
0.02	Reached after one drink
	Feel warm and relaxed
0.05	Talkative and happy
	Lighthearted and giddy
	Lowered inhibitions, judgment, and restraint
	Slightly altered coordination
0.08	Impaired judgment
	Impaired ability to make rational decisions about personal capabilities, such as driving
	Impaired muscle coordination and slowed reaction time
	Numbness of cheeks, lips, arms, and legs
	Tingling of hands, arms, and legs
	Legal impairment in Canada and some U.S. states

BAL (gm/100 ml)	Effects
0.10	Clumsiness and fuzzy speech
	Deterioration of reaction time and muscle control
	Legal intoxication in most states in United States
0.15	Impaired balance and movement
0.2	Slurred speech
	Staggering and loss of balance
	Double vision
0.3	Lack of understanding of what's seen or heard
	Confusion
	Stupor
0.4	Loss of consciousness
	Clammy skin
0.45	Slowed respiration
	Coma
0.5	Breathing may stop; death

Individuals with a long, frequent drinking history develop tolerance to alcohol so that a much higher BAL must be achieved to obtain the effects of a normally lower BAL. I have seen alcoholics walk into the hospital and answer questions reasonably well with BALs above 0.45, a level that would render a nontolerant individual comatose.

Other effects of alcohol include mildly elevated blood pressure; dilation of peripheral blood vessels; increased salivary and gastric secretions; diuresis (excretion of water by the kidneys); sweating; or mild decline in body temperature.

ABSTINENCE SYNDROME

The alcohol abstinence syndrome depends on the frequency and quantity of alcohol ingested, as well as how long the person has been drinking at that level. Typically, it is divided into four stages:

Stage	Signs and symptoms
1	Mild tremor and nervousness
	Nausea
2	Hyperactivity and marked tremor
	Mildly increased body temperature
	Increased startle response
	Mildly increased heart rate and blood pressure
	Insomnia or nightmares when sleep occurs
	Illusions
	Hallucinations (seeing, hearing, or smelling things that aren't there)
3	Same symptoms as stage 2, only more marked
	Grand mal seizures may occur
4	Severe confusion
(delirium	Agitation and insomnia
tremens)	Gross tremor
	Greatly increased heart rate and blood pressure
	Profuse sweating
	Greatly increased body temperature (104 °F or higher)
	Sometimes death, even with good medical care

Fortunately, adolescents rarely, if ever, experience the more severe withdrawal symptoms. The reason for this is unknown.

HEALTH CONSEQUENCES

Alcohol causes the most severe and widespread adverse health consequences of all drugs of abuse, affecting virtually every organ system. Fortunately, many of these require many years of drinking so they are not commonly found in adolescents.

1. *Neurological*
   - Wernicke–Korsakoff syndrome. Wernicke's syndrome consists of nystagmus, which is a rapid uncontrollable

movement of the eyeballs; paralysis of the sixth ocular nerve causing loss of lateral gaze; and ataxia, which is a staggering gait. Korsakoff's syndrome consists of memory loss and confabulation (lying) to cover it up.
- Alcohol dementia: a decline in intellectual functioning.
- Hepatic encephalopathy. This occurs with severe liver disease. Early signs consist of inappropriate behavior, change in sleep habits, and mood swings. It progresses to confusion, disorientation, stupor, and coma.
- Peripheral neuropathy: a burning pain in the feet and legs due to nerve damage.

2. *Gastrointestinal*
   - Fatty liver: fat deposits in the liver.
   - Alcoholic hepatitis: an inflammation of the liver.
   - Cirrhosis: scar tissue replaces normal liver tissue. This eventually leads to enlarged veins in the esophagus (called *varices*) that sometimes bleed profusely, as well as an abdomen full of fluid known as *ascites*.
   - Esophagitis: inflammation of the esophagus. This can progress to stricture.
   - Gastritis: a superficial, widespread inflammation of the stomach wall.
   - Gastric ulcers: deep focal areas of stomach wall destruction.
   - Small intestine: effects such as diarrhea, vitamin deficiencies, and malnutrition.
   - Pancreatitis: inflammation of the pancreas. This condition contributes to malnutrition, diarrhea, and diabetes. It is characterized by nausea, vomiting, and severe abdominal pain.

3. *Cardiovascular*
   - Hypertension: high blood pressure.
   - Cardiomyopathy: damaged heart muscle. This is characterized by congestive heart failure.
   - Cardiac arrhythmias: an irregular heartbeat.

4. *Musculoskeletal*
   - Myopathy: damaged skeletal muscles. This is characterized acutely by weak, swollen, and painful muscles. It is characterized chronically by wasted and weak muscles, particularly in the legs.
   - Aseptic necrosis of the hip: death of the proximal end of leg bone in the hip joint. This occurs due to loss of local blood supply to the bone.
   - Gout: a form of arthritis due to precipitation of uric acid crystals in joints.

5. *Hematological/immunological*
   - Anemia: low red cell count. This is due to blood loss from gastritis or ulcers, poor absorption of vitamins needed to make red blood cells, and the direct depressant effect of alcohol on red blood cell production.
   - Leukopenia: a depressed white blood cell count. This is due to direct suppression of white blood cell production by alcohol. It may lead to various infections.
   - Coagulation disorders: poor blood clotting. This is due to direct suppression of clotting factors and platelet production by alcohol. It can sometimes lead to massive bleeding.
   - Infection: due to a suppressed immune system.

6. *Dermatological*
   - Reddened face and nose.
   - Edematous eyelids and red eyes.
   - Rosacea (rose-red bumps on the face and nose).
   - Scaly skin and seborrhea: this is similar to dandruff but occurs on the face.
   - Cigarette burns.
   - Bruises and ecchymoses: purple areas of skin due to bleeding into the skin.

7. *Nutritional*
   - Nerve and heart problems (beriberi) caused by thiamine deficiency.

- Anemia and inflammation of nerves caused by pyridoxine (vitamin B$_6$) deficiency.
- Diarrhea, dementia, and dermatitis (pellagra) caused by niacin (vitamin B$_3$) deficiency.
- Bleeding into the skin and gum disease (scurvy) caused by vitamin C deficiency.

8. *Cancer*
   - Mouth and esophageal.
   - Pancreas, colon, and rectum (possibly).
   - Stomach, prostate, and thyroid gland (possibly).

CONCLUSIONS

Alcohol is usually abused in the form of either beer, wine, whiskey, or liquor. A 12-ounce can of beer, a 5-ounce glass of wine, and a shot of liquor or whiskey contain approximately the same amount of alcohol.

The effect of alcohol on the brain depends on the blood alcohol level, ranging from feeling warm and relaxed at a very low level to death at a much higher level.

Alcohol withdrawal symptoms range in severity from mild anxiety to delirium tremens and sometimes death, depending on the quantity ingested and the length of time one has been drinking.

Alcohol causes the most severe adverse health consequences of any drug of abuse other than nicotine. The damage can involve virtually every organ system of the body.

Other Depressants

In addition to alcohol, drugs that depress the brain include barbiturates, barbiturate-like drugs, meprobamate, chloral hydrate, and benzodiazepines. These drugs are used mainly to calm and relax (*sedatives*) or to induce sleep (*hypnotics*). Collectively, they are known as *sedative-hypnotics*.

THE DEPRESSANT DRUGS

Barbiturates

A large number of barbiturates are available by prescription. They are classified as ultrashort-acting, short-to-intermediate-acting, and long-acting, based on how long they stay in the body.

Generic name	Trade name
Ultrashort-acting	
methohexital	Brevital
thiopental	Pentothal

Generic name	Trade name
Short-to-intermediate-acting	
amobarbital	Amytal
aprobarbital	Alurate
butabarbital	Butisol
butalbital	Fiorinal, Esgic, Axotal
pentobarbital	Nembutal
secobarbital	Seconal
amobarbital + secobarbital	Tuinal
Long-acting	
mephobarbital	Mebaral
phenobarbital	Luminal

In addition to their sedative and hypnotic effects, some drugs containing barbiturates, such as Fiorinal, Esgic, and Axotal, are used to treat headaches. Others, like Luminal, are used to prevent seizures. Butalbital is available in combination with codeine (Fiorinal #3), also used for the treatment of headaches. Fiorinal #3 supplies the addict with two addicting drugs in one pill.

Barbiturates come in red, yellow, blue, or red and blue capsules and are taken orally.

Barbiturate-like Drugs

The barbiturate-like drugs were developed in an attempt to avoid some of the undesirable side effects of the barbiturates, including their potential for lethal overdose; however, the barbiturate-like drugs can produce tolerance, dependence, and an abstinence syndrome similar to that of the barbiturates. The barbiturate-like drugs are

Generic name	Trade name
ethchlorvynol	Placidyl
ethinamate	Valmid
glutethimide	Doriden
methaqualone	Quaalude
methyprylon	Noludar

Quāāludes are no longer available legally in the United States. The others, although legal by prescription, have very little medical usefulness. All were originally used as hypnotics or sleeping pills. The barbiturate-like drugs come in capsules and tablets and are taken orally.

Meprobamate

Meprobamate, found in drugs such as Equanil and Miltown, at one time was a frequently prescribed sedative. Although still available from physicians, it is seldom prescribed anymore, having been replaced by the benzodiazepines. Meprobamate comes in capsules and is taken orally.

Chloral Hydrate

Chloral hydrate (Noctec) is a hypnotic that, at one time, was widely prescribed for the elderly. It is still available by prescription. Chloral hydrate comes in gelatinous capsules that are taken orally.

Benzodiazepines

Benzodiazepines are among the most widely prescribed drugs in the world. They are divided into short-acting, intermediate-acting, and long-acting groups. They include

Generic name	Trade name
Short-acting	
temazepam	Restoril
triazolam	Halcion

Generic name	Trade name
Intermediate-acting	
alprazolam	Xanax
lorazepam	Ativan
oxazepam	Serax
quazepam	Doral
Long-acting	
chlordiazepoxide	Librium
chlorazepate	Tranxene
clonazepam	Clonopin
diazepam	Valium
flurazepam	Dalmane
halazepam	Paxipam
prazepam	Centrax

Of the benzodiazepines, some, including Restoril, Halcion, Dalmane, and Doral, are hypnotics. The remainder are sedatives. In addition, Valium is prescribed as a muscle relaxant and as a treatment for seizures.

Benzodiazepines are abused as capsules and tablets that are taken orally.

HISTORY

Barbiturates

The first barbiturate, barbital, was synthesized from barbituric acid in 1864, and was first manufactured and used in medicine in 1882. Phenobarbital, a second derivative of barbituric acid, was introduced to the medical profession in 1912 under the trade name of Luminal. In the 1930s, barbiturates were widely prescribed, and in the 1940s the medical communities recognized their potential for abuse and dependence. In the 1950s, barbiturates became some of the most abused drugs in the United States, spreading to adolescents in the 1960s. Despite a decline in popularity, they were still widely prescribed and abused in the 1970s and 1980s. The barbiturates are not commonly prescribed in the 1990s, having been replaced by benzodiazepines (except for butalbital, an ingredient in Fiorinal, Esgic, and Axotal) for headaches, and phenobarbital (Luminal) for seizure prevention. Methaqualone (Quāālude) was first synthesized in India for the treatment of malaria. It was introduced into the United States in 1965 as a treatment for anxiety and insomnia. It was believed to have none of the abuse and dependence properties of the barbiturates. It rapidly became a very popular drug of abuse, however, partly because of the rumor that sex plus a Quāālude was much better than just sex alone. Methaqualone was removed from the market in the 1980s because of its widespread abuse.

Meprobamate

Meprobamate was first synthesized in 1951 as a muscle relaxant. It was subsequently found to have sedative and seizure-prevention properties. It became available in the United States in 1955 and at one time was widely prescribed as a sedative and hypnotic. Although still available by prescription, it has essentially been replaced by benzodiazepines.

Chloral Hydrate

First synthesized in 1869, chloral hydrate was the first totally synthetic sedative-hypnotic. Because it did not cause morning hangover, it was once widely prescribed as a hypnotic for the elderly. It has been depicted in movies as, when added to an alcoholic drink, causing individuals to pass out; hence, the nickname "knock-out drops." The combination of chloral hydrate plus an alcoholic beverage is known as a "Mickey Finn." Chloral hydrate, for the most part, also has been replaced in medicine by the benzodiazepines.

Benzodiazepines

The first benzodiazepine, Librium, was synthesized in 1955 and marketed in 1960. Since that time, the benzodiazepines have become some of the most widely prescribed drugs in the world. In 1971 alone, physicians wrote 50 million prescriptions for Valium and 24 million for Librium, amounting to about $200 million in sales. The use of benzodiazepines in the United States steadily increased through 1975 to a peak level of approximately 100 million prescriptions annually. In the mid-1970s, Valium was the most commonly prescribed drug of any kind. Subsequently, benzodiazepine prescriptions declined to around 50 million. In the past few years, they have been on the rise again. In 1985, 81 million prescriptions for them were filled, and in a household survey, 7.1 percent of adults reported using benzodiazepines. Today, Xanax alone is the fifth most-prescribed medication in the United States.

DRUG CULTURE NAMES

The sedative-hypnotic drugs are known by a variety of names in the drug culture:

Drug	Drug culture names	
Barbiturate		
Amytal	bluebirds	blue tips
	blue devils	blue dolls
	blue heavens	blue bullets
	blues	
Luminal	purple hearts	
Nembutal	nebbies	nimbies
	yellow jackets	yellows
	yellow dolls	yellow bullets
Seconal	reds	red birds
	red devils	Mexican reds
	R. D.	seccies

Drug	Drug culture names	
Babiturates in general	barbs	bears
	blockbusters	downers
	foolpills	goofballs
	green dragons	stumblers
	sleeping pills	
Barbiturate-like drugs		
Quāālude	ludes	quads
	quas	soapers
	sopes	
Doriden	dors and fours (Doriden + codeine)	
Chloral hydrate		
Noctec	Mickey Finn (chloral hydrate + alcohol)	
	knockout drops (chloral hydrate + alcohol)	

ACTIONS

The sedative-hypnotic drugs produce

- sedation
- hypnosis
- suppressed REM sleep (that part of sleep that is associated with dreaming)
- confusion and disorientation
- slurred speech
- difficulty in thinking
- impaired psychomotor performance
- slowness of speech and comprehension
- dizziness and ataxia
- poor memory
- faulty judgment
- a narrowed range of attention

These effects should be recognized as the same as those produced by alcohol. I often tell patients that the brain can't tell the difference between a shot of liquor and a Valium tablet.

ABSTINENCE SYNDROME

The sedative-hypnotic drugs, on cessation of abuse, can cause almost identical withdrawal symptoms as alcohol. Withdrawal symptoms include

- anxiety, insomnia, and panic attacks
- tremor and hyperactive reflexes
- nausea and vomiting
- elevated blood pressure
- agitation, irritability, and sweating
- increased heart rate
- seizures
- confusion and delirium
- psychosis
- drug craving

The combination of delirium and psychosis very much resembles delirium tremens (DTs).

The benzodiazepine abstinence syndrome can produce an especially troublesome problem. A small percentage of people who take them as prescribed for over three months become seriously addicted to them. These unfortunate individuals have waxing and waning withdrawal symptoms, including anxiety, panic attacks, and insomnia, that last up to six months after cessation of use. Some even have one or more seizures. Benzodiazepine use should never be stopped suddenly. Instead, the dose should be tapered over 6 to 12 weeks. Physicians, in general, have not given benzodiazepines the respect they deserve. They are learning, however, that these drugs are addicting and that they can produce serious withdrawal symptoms.

HEALTH CONSEQUENCES

All sedative-hypnotics in overdose can produce

- shallow breathing, respiratory arrest

- hypotension (a lowering of the blood pressure) and circulatory collapse
- aspiration pneumonia (inhaling one's own vomitus)
- depressed heart function
- hypothermia (a reduced body temperature)
- stupor, coma
- death

The benzodiazepines are safer than the other sedative-hypnotics in that much larger doses are required to produce the above effects.

Adverse health consequences from long-term benzodiazepine use are not known, except for depression, which has, in some individuals, lead to suicide.

CONCLUSIONS

In addition to alcohol, drugs that depress the functioning of the brain include barbiturates, barbiturate-like drugs, meprobamate, chloral hydrate, and benzodiazepines. These drugs are used mainly to calm and relax (sedatives) or to induce sleep (hypnotics). Collectively, they are known as sedative-hypnotics. They produce the same effects on the brain as alcohol, and their abstinence syndromes are similar to that of alcohol.

22

Opioids

The term *opioid* is used to designate a group of drugs that are morphine-like in their actions. Because of the fact that opioid drugs tend to sedate, they are often referred to as *narcotics*, a word that comes from *narcosis* (meaning sleep). Because they also produce euphoria, opioid drugs are often abused. Opioids are commonly used in medicine to reduce pain, as cough suppressants, and to control diarrhea.

Narcotic addicts will go to extremes to get opioid drugs, including faking medical problems. Faking a kidney stone is a common act. Addicts may even prick their fingers with pins to add drops of blood to their urine samples to fool the laboratories. They commonly go away with prescriptions for very powerful narcotics.

An addict acquainted with the author would go from one emergency department to another faking symptoms of a heart attack. He was exceptionally good at it, and invariably was admitted to coronary care unit after coronary care unit where he had his "chest pain" treated with intravenous morphine.

Narcotic addicts have been known to fake medical problems requiring abdominal surgery to get drugs.

THE OPIOID DRUGS

Opioid drugs are classified as (1) naturally occurring, (2) semi-synthetic, (3) synthetic, and (4) agonist–antagonist.

Naturally Occurring Opioids

The naturally occurring opioids are extracted directly from the poppy plant (*Papaver somniferum*). They include

Generic name	Selected trade names	Medical use
opium	Paregoric	diarrhea
	Parepectolin	diarrhea
	Pantopon	pain
	B & O Supprettes	pain
	Donnagel-PG	diarrhea
morphine	Morphine sulfate	pain, pulmonary edema, adjunct to anesthesia
	Duramorph	pain
	Roxanol	pain
codeine	Empirin with codeine	pain
	Tylenol with codeine	pain
	Phenergan with codeine	cough
	Robitussin AC	cough

Opium comes as dark brown chunks or powders. It can be smoked, eaten, or injected. Morphine comes as white crystals, tablets, or injected solutions. It is taken orally, injected, or snorted. Codeine comes as a dark liquid (varying in thickness), capsules, and tablets. It is taken orally or injected.

Semisynthetic Opioids

The semisynthetic opioids are drugs that are made by the pharmaceutical industry by relatively simple modifications of the morphine molecule. They include

Generic name	Trade name	Medical use
heroin	none	none
hydrocodone	Hycodan	cough
	Hycomine	cough
	Tussionex	cough
	Lorcet-HD	pain
	Vicodin	pain
hydromorphone	Dilaudid	pain
oxycodone	Percodan	pain
	Percocet	pain
	Tylox	pain

Heroin comes as a white- to dark-brown powder or a tar-like substance. It is a very versatile drug. It can be smoked, snorted, or injected subcutaneously (under the skin), intramuscularly, or intravenously. Intravenous injection, however, is its main route of use. In many areas of the country, heroin has been replaced for the most part by Dilaudid, a very powerful legal drug that is diverted to the drug culture for illegal use. The tablets are ground up, dissolved in water, and injected intravenously. Heroin, however, in a very potent form, seems to be making a comeback.

Tussionex, used medically for cough, and Percodan, a pain medication, are particularly popular drugs of abuse.

Other semisynthetic narcotics such as Hycodan, Lorcet HD, Vicodin, Tylox, and Percocet come as tablets. They are taken orally.

Synthetic Opioids

The synthetic opioids are synthesized in the laboratory totally independent of the poppy plant. They include

Generic name	Trade name	Medical use
alphaprodine	Nisentil	pain (obstetrical)
diphenoxylate	Lomotil	diarrhea
fentanyl	Sublimaze	pain, adjunct to anesthesia

Generic name	Trade name	Medical use
levorphanol	Levo-Dromoran	pain
loperamide	Imodium	diarrhea
meperidine	Demerol	pain
methadone	Dolophine	pain, maintenance of narcotic dependence
propoxyphene	Darvon	pain
	Darvon-N	pain
	SK-65	pain
	Wygesic	pain

Methadone is primarily used in methadone maintenance clinics in larger cities where heroin addiction is a major problem. Basically, heroin addicts are given methadone free of charge on a daily basis to replace heroin use in an attempt to reduce criminal activity and to improve their family and community functioning. In addition, since it is taken orally in the form of tablets or liquid rather than injected, methadone maintenance also serves to reduce the rates of serious infections, such as hepatitis and AIDS. Since methadone is an opioid, the purpose of methadone maintenance is not to produce drug-free individuals. Methadone, itself, is sometimes abused.

Sublimaze comes in an injectable liquid. It is sometimes abused by anesthesiologists and nurse anesthetists.

Demerol comes in a white powder, tablets and vials. It is taken orally and injected. It is sometimes abused by nurses.

Other synthetic narcotics, such as Nisentil and Levo-dromoran, come in vials and are injected. Others, like Lomotil, Imodium, Darvon, Darvon-N, Lorcet, SK-65, and Wygesic, come in tablets and are taken orally.

Agonist–Antagonist Opioids

The agonist–antagonist opioid drugs include

Generic name	Trade name	Medical use
buprenorphine	Buprenex	pain
butorphanol	Stadol	pain
nalbuphine	Nubain	pain
pentazocine	Talwin	pain

Of this group of drugs, Talwin has been the most abused. Most often, the tablets are ground up, dissolved in water, and injected intravenously in combination with an antihistamine (pyribenzamine), which is thought by addicts to increase Talwin's psychoactive effects. The combination is known as "Ts and blues" in the drug culture.

Other synthetic narcotics, such as Buprenex, Stadol, and Nubain, come in tablets and vials, and are taken orally or injected. Buprenex is currently being investigated for its apparent ability to decrease cocaine craving.

Designer Opioids

Designer drugs are substances that are illegally developed in basement laboratories and which have structures and properties similar to those of scheduled drugs. There have been two designer opioids—fentanyl analogues and meperidine analogues.

Fentanyl Analogues

In drug culture mythology, "China white" is an extremely potent form of heroin that produces the perfect high. Designer fentanyl drugs became associated with this myth, and have become known as China white. A number of fentanyl analogues have been developed, ranging in potency from 200 to 1000 times as powerful as morphine. Because of their extreme potency, several overdose deaths have accidentally occurred. Most recently, a designer fentanyl known as "Tango and Cash" has been responsible for a number of deaths in the Northeast. Most of these deaths occurred in the home. Some addicts were reportedly found dead with the needles still in their arms.

Meperidine Analogues

In 1982, Parkinson-like symptoms (muscle rigidity, tremor, and paralysis) began showing up in California addicts who had injected a drug they called synthetic heroin. The drug was supposed to have been a designer Demerol (MPPP). Instead, due to sloppy basement chemistry, the drug that was produced was MPTP, which destroyed brain cells in a part of the brain called the substantia nigra, interfering with dopamine synthesis and, thus, accounting for the symptoms.

HISTORY

Opium

Opium is made by air-drying the juice of the unripe seed pods of the Oriental poppy, and has been used since ancient times. The first recorded use dates back to 5000 BC in Mesopotamia. It was used in 1500 BC as an anesthetic by Egyptian physicians, and in the Middle East in 1200 AD as a medicine and intoxicant. A tincture of opium (laudanum) was used as early as 1541 to relieve pain, to treat dysentery, to suppress cough, and to sedate.

By 1560, opium smoking had become a major problem in China. As a result, the Chinese government tried to control its importation, sale, and use. The British opposed this because it interfered with their profitable trade of opium grown in India. This led to the Opium Wars (1835–1842), which the British won. As a result, the practice continued and led to the importation of opium to the United States and elsewhere by Chinese immigrants.

During the 1870s, patent medicines containing opium proliferated. The most important of these was paregoric, a tincture of opium combined with camphor, still used today to control diarrhea. The Harrison Narcotic Act in 1914 placed opium under strict federal control, and the Controlled Substance Act in 1970 placed it in Schedule II.

Morphine

Morphine, the principle psychoactive ingredient of opium, was extracted from the plant in 1803 and named for Morpheus, the god of sleep and dreams. When morphine was introduced to the medical profession in 1825, it was touted not only as a powerful pain medication, but also as a cure for opium addiction, which, of course, turned out to be far from the truth. Invention of the hypodermic needle in 1853 made possible almost immediate relief of pain, and physicians prescribed morphine liberally. It could be purchased from the local drugstore or ordered by mail without a prescription, as could hypodermic needles.

During the Civil War (1861–1865), morphine was used liberally for anesthesia and pain relief, and soldiers were given the drug as well as hypodermic needles for use when they returned home. It has been estimated that as many as 400,000 morphine addicts were created in this manner. Morphine was synthesized independently of the poppy plant in 1925, and continues to be used as a major drug in medicine for relief of severe pain, treatment of pulmonary edema (excess fluid in the lungs), and as an adjunct to anesthesia.

Heroin

Heroin was first derived from morphine in 1874 and produced commercially by the Bayer pharmaceutical company in 1898. Its name comes from the German word *heroisch*, meaning powerful. Heroin rapidly replaced opium and morphine as the major drug of abuse in the United States. In 1924, its manufacture was prohibited; however, it rapidly became available on the black market, smuggled in from Southeast Asia and Mexico.

DRUG CULTURE NAMES

The opioid drugs are known by a variety of names in the drug culture.

Generic name	Drug culture names	
opium	O	gum
	op	hop
	black pills	tar
	black stuff	blue velvet (paregoric)
morphine	M	dreamer
	morph	Miss Emma
	M.S.	
codeine	schoolboys	pops
heroin	H	smack
	big H	white stuff
	horse	thing
	Harry	duster (heroin + tobacco)
	junk	A-bomb (heroin + marijuana)
	joy powder	speedball (heroin + cocaine)
	Mexican brown	mud
hydromorphone	fours	dillies
	D	lords
methadone	dollies	wafers
	dolls	10-8-20
propoxyphene	pinks and grays	
pentazocine	Ts and blues (Talwin + pyribenzamine)	
fentanyl	China white	Tango and Cash

ACTIONS

Opioids have a multitude of actions on the body.

1. *Brain*
   - reduced pain
   - drowsiness and sedation
   - ataxia and impaired coordination
   - nausea and vomiting
   - euphoria
   - impaired reflexes
   - dizziness and syncope (passing out)
   - miosis (constricted pupils)
2. *Cardiovascular*
   - dilation of peripheral blood vessels
3. *Respiratory*
   - decreased breathing rate and depth
4. *Gastrointestinal*
   - decreased propulsive movements of the intestines
5. *Genitourinary*
   - increased tone of urinary bladder wall and sphincter
   - decreased tone of uterus during labor

ABSTINENCE SYNDROME

The opioid abstinence syndrome can be extremely uncomfortable, but it is not life-threatening, except to unborn fetuses. It consists of

- rhinorrhea (runny nose) and lacrimation (tearing)
- yawning
- chills and goose pimples
- hyperventilation
- hypothermia (lowered body temperature)
- increased heart rate
- mydriasis (dilated pupils)
- muscle aches and spasms
- bone pain

- nausea, vomiting, and diarrhea
- anxiety, hostility, and insomnia
- opioid craving

The acute abstinence syndrome runs its course in four to five days for most opioid drugs. Methadone withdrawal, however (because the drug stays in the body a long time), may take up to two weeks. The postacute abstinence syndrome lasts several months and is characterized by many of the symptoms listed above but at a much lower level of intensity.

HEALTH CONSEQUENCES

The two major health consequences of opioid abuse are infections and overdose. Infections from opioid injection include

- cellulitis (a superficial skin infection) and skin abscesses
- thrombophlebitis (an infection of veins)
- endocarditis (a heart valve infection)
- brain and lung abscesses
- hepatitis B (a viral liver infection)
- AIDS

Overdose can result in

- depression of breathing
- pulmonary edema (excess fluid in the lungs)
- hypotension (a drop in blood pressure)
- circulatory collapse
- death

Other effects include a decreased libido, amenorrhea (lack of menstrual period), and chronic constipation. These symptoms resolve themselves when opioid use is stopped.

CONCLUSIONS

Opioids, also called narcotics, are drugs that are morphine-like in their actions. They are used in medicine to reduce pain, relieve cough, and control diarrhea. They are often abused.

Potent designer opioids have been illegally manufactured and sold. Some of these have resulted in disastrous medical consequences for the user.

Unlike delirium tremens, the opioid abstinence syndrome, although extremely unpleasant, is not life-threatening.

The primary health consequences of opioid abuse are infections at various sites (skin, heart valves, liver) and death from accidental overdose.

Cocaine

THE FORMS OF COCAINE

Cocaine comes from the *Erythroxylon* coca plant. The drug can be used in several forms: coca leaves, coca paste, cocaine hydrochloride, freebase cocaine, and rock or crack cocaine. The only medical use of cocaine is as a topical anesthetic, and as a vasoconstrictor in nasal surgery. By constricting blood vessels cocaine reduces tissue swelling and makes it easier for physicians to see into the nose.

Coca Leaves

Coca leaves are toasted, mixed with alkaline ash from other burned leaves, and chewed. The alkaline material improves absorption into the blood vessels of the mouth. Chewing coca leaves is a relatively safe practice because the leaves contain only 0.5 to 1 percent cocaine. Although absorption is initially effective, the local constriction of blood vessels, which reduces local blood flow, slows absorption. Coca leaf chewing is a practice limited to the Indians of the Andes Mountains in South America.

Coca Paste

Coca paste is made by mixing coca leaves with gasoline, kerosene, or sulfuric acid to produce a crude paste that is smoked in cigarette form in South America. It can be dangerous to one's health because of the impurities it contains.

Cocaine Hydrochloride

This is the purified form of cocaine, which is extracted from coca paste with hydrochloric acid, and is a white, crystalline powder. It is smuggled into the United States in pure form and then cut with a variety of agents to dilute the cocaine. Cocaine hydrochloride can be swallowed or used intranasally or intravenously. It cannot be smoked because it does not volatilize sufficiently.

When used orally, 70 to 80 percent of cocaine hydrochloride is inactivated during its first pass through the liver on the way from the intestine to the bloodstream.

When snorted, cocaine is placed on a hard surface such as a mirror, chopped with a razor blade to remove lumps, and made into lines. The lines are then snorted through a straw or a rolled-up bill. Intranasal cocaine hydrochloride constricts blood vessels in the nose, limiting its own absorption. Because of the more rapid onset of its action and greater peak blood level achieved by this route, snorting cocaine is more addicting than coca leaf chewing or oral cocaine use.

Intravenous injection of cocaine hydrochloride delivers 100 percent of the drug to the bloodstream. The quicker onset, shorter duration of action and the higher blood level achieved with this route make intravenous administration much more addicting than the intranasal route.

Freebase Cocaine

With the aid of a volatile substance such as ether, the base form of cocaine hydrochloride can be freed and is called *freebase cocaine*; it is smoked. This is a highly addictive form of cocaine, even more so than intravenously injected cocaine. Freebasing cocaine can be a dangerous process. Serious burns have occurred. As a result, its popularity has waned.

Rock or Crack Cocaine

The most popular form, rock or crack cocaine, is produced by mixing cocaine hydrochloride with baking soda and heating it. Because the end result is small pieces of material that resemble rocks, it is called *rock cocaine*. Because rock cocaine makes a crackling sound when it is smoked, it is also known as *crack cocaine*. It is another form of freebase cocaine.

Crack cocaine comes as white to tan pellets, or crystalline rocks that look like soap. It also is smoked.

How Crack Cocaine Is Used

The most popular method of using crack cocaine is to smoke it in a pipe, but sometimes it is smoked by sprinkling it on tobacco or marijuana. It is frequently used with a depressant drug, usually alcohol or Valium, to moderate the irritability it causes. Because its effects last only a few minutes, its use must be repeated about every 20 minutes to maintain the euphoria and avoid the crash. This often leads to a run that lasts for several days until the addict runs out of the drug or collapses from exhaustion. During the run, he does not eat, sleep, or have sex. His only interest is using the cocaine. Patients have been known to spend their savings, sell their car, and steal from their parents to keep a run going. The desire to use the drug can be overwhelming.

HISTORY

Cocaine has been used for its stimulant effects for hundreds of years. The coca plant was originally found along the Andes Mountains in Bolivia and Peru. Andes Indians chewed coca leaves, and from the 11th to 15th centuries (during the reign of the Incas), popular myths considered it to be of divine origin—a gift from the sun god.

When the Spaniards conquered the Incas in the 16th century, they banned the use of coca leaves; however, they soon found they couldn't get the Incas to work in the mines and fields without it. As a result, the Catholic church, for a period of time, became the largest grower of coca plants in South America.

Cocaine did not become popular in Europe at that time because it lost most of its potency during the long voyage from the New World. In 1859, Alfred Niemann solved this problem by extracting the pure substance from the plant. He named it cocaine.

Sigmund Freud, the father of modern psychiatry, experimented with the use of cocaine, and also prescribed it to his patients for a variety of psychiatric disorders. He discontinued the practice when one of his colleagues became a cocaine addict and one of his patients died of an overdose.

Robert Louis Stevenson is said to have written *Dr. Jekyll and Mr. Hyde* during a three-day cocaine binge, giving you some idea of what going on and coming off cocaine was like for him.

At the turn of the century, Coca-Cola and several patent medicines containing cocaine were marketed. Coca wine, called Vin Mariani, gave the user both alcohol and cocaine. Because of widespread cocaine addiction, cocaine was replaced in Coca-Cola by another stimulant, caffeine, in 1906.

Because of rampant abuse, cocaine was banned by the Harrison Narcotic Act of 1914. Its use thereafter greatly declined.

In the late 1960s and early 1970s, cocaine use reemerged. Its primary route of administration was intranasal. In the late 1970s and early 1980s, the use of freebase cocaine spread rapidly, and in the mid-1980s, crack cocaine became the predominant form of cocaine abused. As a result of its highly addictive nature, the number of people addicted to crack cocaine increased rapidly, and has now reached epidemic proportions. Cocaine is currently the largest source of illicit drug income in the United States.

DRUG CULTURE NAMES

Cocaine is known by a variety of names by its users. Many of these names reflect how addicts feel about the drug:

base	line
C	nose candy
coca	nose powder
coke	paradise
crack	rock
freebase	snow
girl	speedball (cocaine + heroin)
heaven dust	toot
lady	the champagne of drugs

ACTIONS

The actions of cocaine depend on whether the person has just begun using it, known as acute use, or has been using it a long period of time, known as chronic use.

Acute Use
- Euphoria and grandiosity
- Feelings of enhanced sexuality
- Feelings of enhanced mental capacity
- Increased sociability

- Decreased fatigue and increased energy
- Anorexia (loss of appetite)
- Indifference to pain
- Dilated pupils

Chronic Use

- Dysphoria (depression)
- Sexual disinterest, impotence
- Irritability, anxiety, insomnia
- Weight loss and personal neglect
- Inability to concentrate
- Visual hallucinations
- Tactile hallucinations ("coke bugs"): feeling bugs that aren't there crawling on your skin
- Suspiciousness
- Delusions (false ideas believed to be true)
- Paranoid psychosis: severely out of touch with reality and believing that others are out to get you

Other effects of cocaine include increased heart rate, blood pressure, and breathing rate, as well as hyperactive reflexes.

Paranoid psychosis is a particularly troubling symptom of prolonged cocaine use. Its signs and symptoms are identical to those of paranoid schizophrenia. Psychiatrists cannot tell the difference unless it occurs to them to get a urine drug screen. I had one patient who blew away the front door of his parents' house with a shotgun because he thought somebody was trying to get in to kill him. Another shot the ceiling of her family's home full of holes with a pistol because she thought "something" in the attic was trying to get her.

ABSTINENCE SYNDROME

The cocaine abstinence syndrome consists of

- Negativism and pessimism
- Irritability and lack of patience

- Fatigue and sleepiness
- Hunger
- Depression
- Intense cocaine craving

The depression is described as *anhedonia*, which is an inability to obtain pleasure in life. The anhedonia, which may last two to three months, is dangerous because it may contribute to relapse. The cocaine abstinence syndrome, as a rule, does not require treatment with medication. The prolonged depression, however, may respond to antidepressant therapy.

HEALTH CONSEQUENCES

Many of the health consequences of cocaine abuse are related to the route of administration. Snorting cocaine affects mainly the nose, causing such problems as:

- rhinitis (inflammation of the lining of the nose)
- nasal bleeding
- nasal mucosa atrophy (thinning of the lining of the nasal passages)
- sinusitis (inflammation of the sinuses)
- hoarseness
- difficulty swallowing
- nasal septal perforation: a hole in the cartilage separating the right side of the nose from the left

Smoking cocaine affects primarily the lungs, causing

- chronic cough
- bronchitis (inflammation of the airways)
- hemoptysis (coughing up blood)
- impaired lung function
- pulmonary edema (excessive fluid in the lungs)

Injecting cocaine intravenously, due to "dirty" needles, leads primarily to infection problems:

- infection at the local injection site, such as abscesses or cellulitis
- hepatitis B (serum hepatitis, a viral liver infection)
- bacterial endocarditis (infection of the heart valves)
- sepsis (spread of an infection throughout the body)
- AIDS (acquired immune deficiency syndrome)

Cocaine by any route can lead to:

- vitamin deficiencies
- anorexia and weight loss
- sexual dysfunction
- cardiac arrhythmias (irregular heartbeat)
- myocardial infarction (heart attack)
- stroke

CONCLUSIONS

Cocaine, a powerful stimulant, is used in several forms in the United States: cocaine hydrochloride, freebase cocaine, and rock or crack cocaine. Cocaine hydrochloride is a white powder that is smuggled into the United States from South America. It is snorted or injected intravenously. Freebase cocaine, which is smoked, is produced from cocaine hydrochloride by a dangerous process that uses ether. Crack or rock cocaine is produced by mixing cocaine hydrochloride with baking soda and heating it, usually in a microwave oven. It is smoked and is highly addictive.

The cocaine abstinence syndrome is rather mild and not life-threatening.

Many of the health consequences of cocaine abuse are the result of the route of administration—intranasal, intravenous, or inhaled. Cocaine by any route can cause heart attacks, irregular heart beats, strokes, and death.

24

Nicotine

THE NICOTINE DRUGS

The most common form of nicotine addiction is cigarette smoking; however, nicotine addiction to a lesser extent is also associated with cigar and pipe smoking, as well as with the use of smokeless tobacco (snuff and chewing tobacco).

There are approximately 3.7 million teenage smokers—about 16 percent of all teenagers. The majority of them claim they expect to quit smoking within a year. Three out of four will fail. They greatly underestimate the addictiveness of nicotine and greatly overestimate their ability to control it.

Among youths with at least two smoking friends, nearly one-half are smokers, whereas among youths with no smoking friends, only 3 percent smoke. Teenagers are three times as likely to smoke if family members smoke. The most influential family members are older brothers and sisters. In homes where older siblings smoke, 30 percent of the younger siblings smoke compared with 15 percent of teenagers from homes where only the parents smoke.

According to Dupont, adolescents who smoke are twice as likely to use alcohol, nine times as likely to use depressant and stimulant drugs, ten times as likely to smoke marijuana, and fourteen times as likely to use cocaine, opioids, and hallucinogens. For this reason, nicotine is often referred to as a *gateway drug*.

HISTORY

The oldest cited evidence of tobacco use appears on a Mayan stone carving dated 600–900 AD. When Columbus discovered the New World in 1492, the Indians offered him dried tobacco leaves as a friendly gesture. He observed the natives inhaling smoke from a hollow reed as part of their religious ceremony. They called the reed *tabacum*, from which our word *tobacco* comes. Tobacco was taken back to Europe by Columbus's crew. The smoke from this early tobacco was harsh and irritating.

Tobacco use spread throughout the rest of the world in the 16th and 17th centuries. In 1604, King James I condemned its use and taxed it heavily. He used the tax money to build fleets for further exploration of the New World.

Opponents of tobacco attributed increased crime, nervous paralysis, loss of intellectual ability, and visual impairment to its use. Others felt tobacco, in the form of poultices and extracts, to be a cure for every known affliction, including cancer.

John Rolfe, an early colonist, developed a tobacco with a milder smoke. This increased the demand for tobacco. His marriage to Pocahontas established peace with the Indians and allowed production to increase to meet the new demand. Sir Walter Raleigh experimented with planting methods and methods of curing tobacco, resulting in an ever milder smoke.

The Egyptians are credited with the development of the modern cigarette. They began wrapping tobacco in paper around 1832. French and British soldiers took these paper-wrapped cylinders back to Europe in 1856 following the Crimean War. Soon after this, cigarettes made their way to the United States.

James Bonsack, a young Virginia inventor, devised a machine in 1881 for mass producing cigarettes. This reduced the price, thus greatly increasing usage.

Manufacturers began to add filters in the early part of the 20th century, primarily to increase the appeal to women, who objected to getting tobacco stains on their fingers. Following the Surgeon General's 1964 report, which publicized some of the health consequences of smoking, the tobacco industry introduced a variety of more functional filters.

In the mid 1960s, 42 percent of adults smoked—52 percent of men and 34 percent of women. By 1988 this had fallen to 26.5 percent—29.5 percent of men and 23.8 percent of women. If these trends continue, by the year 2000 more women than men will smoke. Already, more adolescent girls smoke than boys.

ACTIONS

As a drug, nicotine produces a variety of effects:

- Stimulation of the brain
- Decreased strength of stomach contractions
- Elevated blood pressure
- Increased heart rate
- Dilation of blood vessels
- Reduction of growth hormone secretion—smoking does stunt your growth
- Decreased muscle tone

ABSTINENCE SYNDROME

Nicotine withdrawal symptoms very much resemble those of cocaine and other stimulant drugs:

- Decreased heart rate
- Restlessness, irritability, and hostility
- Dullness or sleepiness
- Inability to concentrate
- Sleep disturbances

- Constipation or diarrhea
- Weight gain
- Nicotine craving

After suddenly stopping smoking, withdrawal symptoms occur within a few hours and last up to three weeks, except for the craving, which may last for months.

HEALTH CONSEQUENCES

Cigarette smoke is composed of hundreds of substances. The harmful effects are produced primarily by carbon monoxide and tars, as well as the nicotine itself. The carbon monoxide combines competitively with the hemoglobin in blood, displacing oxygen. The blood, therefore, is less able to deliver oxygen to the tissues of the body. The tars contain the carcinogens, or cancer-producing substances. Nicotine, in addition to being the drug that produces addiction, also raises the LDL-cholesterol (bad cholesterol) and lowers the HDL-cholesterol (good cholesterol), thereby increasing the risk of atherosclerosis and cardiovascular disease. The health consequences of cigarette smoking are divided into those resulting from active smoking (the smoker) and those resulting from passive smoking (nonsmokers who inhale the smoke of others). In addition, the use of smokeless tobacco produces some adverse health consequences.

Active Smoking

It is estimated that as many as 390,000 deaths a year in the United States may be attributed to cigarette smoking. This represents 18 percent of all deaths. Lung cancer is now the number one cause of cancer death in women as well as men. Lung cancer surpassed breast cancer deaths in women in 1986. Numerous diseases and conditions are associated with cigarette smoking:

1. *Cancer*
   - mouth and throat
   - esophagus
   - lung
   - pancreas
   - kidney and bladder
2. *Cardiovascular*
   - aggravation of exercise-induced angina (heart pain)
   - coronary artery disease
   - myocardial infarction (heart attack)
   - cardiac arrhythmias (irregular heart beat)
   - stroke
   - aortic aneurysm (ballooning of the major artery coming from the heart)
   - Buerger's disease (constriction of blood vessels supplying the hands in response to cold)
3. *Pulmonary*
   - emphysema (destruction of the small air sacs of the lungs)
   - acute and chronic bronchitis (inflammation of the airways)
   - chronic cough
   - vocal cord irritation and hoarseness
4. *Perinatal effects (maternal smoking)*
   - increased infant mortality rate
   - reduced birth weight
   - spontaneous abortion
   - sudden infant death syndrome (SIDS)
   - birth defects
   - hyperactivity in childhood
   - risk of cancer later in life
5. *Miscellaneous*
   - peptic ulcers
   - smoker's skin (early wrinkling)
   - decreased sense of taste and smell

- decreased growth rate
- decreased sperm counts
- decreased fertility
- altered metabolism of some medications
- adverse cardiovascular events in women taking oral contraceptive pills

Passive Smoking

It has been estimated that as many as 53,000 deaths a year in the United States result from passive smoking. In addition, out of the 5000 deaths a year from fires inadvertently set by cigarette smokers, 2000 victims are nonsmokers. Other health consequences from breathing another's smoke include:

1. *Cancer*
   - lung

2. *Cardiovascular*
   - aggravation of exercise-induced angina (heart pain)
   - premature ventricular beats (premature contractions of the large chambers of the heart)

3. *Pulmonary*
   - asthma attacks
   - lung and airway infections
   - bronchiolitis (constriction of airways in infants)
   - decreased growth rate of the lungs in children

4. *Perinatal (paternal smoking)*
   - decreased birth weight, although not as much as with maternal smoking

5. *Miscellaneous*
   - increased hospital admissions of infants, primarily for respiratory infections
   - middle ear infections in children
   - sinusitis in children

- decreased growth rate (even passive smoking stunts children's growth to a degree)

Smokeless Tobacco

Health consequences from smokeless tobacco result primarily from local action of the cancer-producing agents in tobacco. Precancerous lesions in the mouth are common in young chewing tobacco users. Many of these lesions progress to cancer if the practice continues. In addition, nicotine, absorbed in the mouth and distributed throughout the body by the blood, produces the effects previously mentioned.

TREATMENT OF NICOTINE ADDICTION

Adolescents who use tobacco products should be urged to quit. If they are unable to do so by themselves, help is available. The most effective method consists of setting a quit date, detoxification with a nicotine transdermal system (patch) to minimize withdrawal symptoms, and behavioral modification to help them quit and stay that way. Nicotine patches contain a fixed amount of nicotine that is released in a controlled manner, crossing the skin and entering the bloodstream when applied to the skin. A new patch is applied daily and the old one removed. After a few weeks, a smaller patch is used for a few more weeks. Then a final patch, yet smaller, is applied for a few more weeks. In this way, a person receives a tapering dose of nicotine.

Behavioral modification consists of steps to take prior to the quitting date and steps to take after the quitting date.

Steps Prior to the Quit Date

The following steps should be taken prior to the actual act of quitting:

- Waiting ten minutes before smoking after an urge to do so.
- Buying cigarettes by the single pack only.
- Not smoking in the car.
- Smoking the least pleasurable brand.
- Cutting down to a pack per day if more than this is smoked.
- Thinking about quitting one day at a time, not for the rest of one's life.
- Making a list of the times, places, and situations in which the urge to smoke is greatest.
- Having smoked the last cigarette the evening prior to the quit date, throw away all cigarettes, cigarette lighters, and ashtrays, and apply the first patch.

Steps to Take after the Quit Date

The following steps can be taken after the quit date:

- Taking five deep breaths and exhaling slowly after each when an urge to smoke occurs.
- Playing with a pen to occupy the hand that usually has a cigarette in it.
- Sucking air through a cut-off soda straw when the urge to smoke is particularly strong.
- Rubbing the patch gently and saying softly, "This is all the nicotine I need" when an urge to smoke occurs.
- Playing a relaxation tape from time to time if one tends to smoke when anxious.
- Avoiding the times, places, and situations in which the urge to smoke is greatest, or making plans about how to deal with them if they can't be avoided.

If one has tried to stop smoking and failed, the next step is to locate a physician who is actively involved in the treatment of nicotine addiction. All physicians can write prescriptions for the patches, but not all give the behavioral modification support that many patients need.

CONCLUSIONS

Nicotine is a stimulant drug. The most common form of addiction to it is cigarette smoking. Nicotine withdrawal symptoms very much resemble those of cocaine.

The health consequences of cigarette smoking, both active and passive, are numerous and involve most organ systems of the body. Cigarette smoking is the leading preventable cause of premature death in the United States today.

Treatment of nicotine addiction is effective for many and is readily available. Nicotine patches and behavioral modification is currently the treatment of choice.

25

Other Stimulants

Other stimulant drugs include amphetamines, amphetamine co-geners, caffeine, methylphenidate, and phenylpropanolamine.

THE STIMULANT DRUGS

Amphetamines

The amphetamines are prescription drugs sometimes used for the treatment of obesity, attention deficit disorder (hyperactive child syndrome), and narcolepsy (inability to stay awake). They are Schedule II drugs. Illicit amphetamines are manufactured in basement laboratories. The amphetamines include:

Generic name	Trade name
amphetamine sulfate	Benzedrine
dextroamphetamine	Dexedrine
methamphetamine	Desoxyn
dextroamphetamine + amphetamine sulfate	Biphetamine

Amphetamine comes as capsules or tablets that are taken orally. Methamphetamine comes as a white powder, tablets, or rocks that resemble blocks of paraffin. It is taken orally, smoked, or injected.

Amphetamine Cogeners

The amphetamine cogeners are prescription diet pills. They include:

Generic name	Trade name
benzphetamine	Didrex
diethylpropion	Tenuate, Tepanil
fenfluramine	Pondimin
mazindol	Mazanor, Sanorex
phendimetrazine	Plegine, Prelu-2, Trimstat
phenmetrazine	Preludin
phenterine	Fastin, Adipex-P, Teramine

The amphetamine cogeners are classified in Schedules II, III, or IV, depending on their potential for abuse and dependence. Because at one time these drugs were widely abused, the American Medical Association discourages their routine prescribing.

Amphetamine cogeners come as tablets and capsules that are taken orally.

Methylphenidate

Methylphenidate (Ritalin) is a weaker stimulant than the amphetamines, and thus it has less potential for abuse and dependence. It is the medication of choice for most children with attention deficit disorder, and for the treatment of narcolepsy. In sufficient doses, however, it can produce the same effects as amphetamines. Ritalin comes as tablets that are taken orally.

The author has only seen two cases of adult Ritalin abuse. In each case, a child in the family was taking prescribed Ritalin for hyperactive behavior. The parents began abusing the drug, primarily because of its ready availability.

Phenylpropanolamine

Phenylpropanolamine is a common ingredient in many prescription and over-the-counter medications. It is a weak stimulant that is often misrepresented in the drug culture and sold as amphetamines. It is the most common ingredient in over-the-counter diet pills (Acutrim, Appedrine, Dexatrim, Ordinex) in which it may be combined with another stimulant such as caffeine. Being a decongestant, it is also a common ingredient in over-the-counter cold, cough, and allergy medications such as Allerest, Alka Seltzer Plus, Contac, Coricidin-D, Naldecon, and Sinarest.

Phenylpropanolamine comes as tablets and capsules that are taken orally. It is not a benign drug. Taken in sufficient quantity, it can have the same effects as amphetamines.

Caffeine

Caffeine is found in many plants throughout the world. It is an ingredient in coffee, tea, and carbonated soft drinks. It is also an ingredient in many over-the-counter cold medications, headache remedies, diet pills, and stimulants such as Vivarin and NoDoz, as well as in many prescription headache preparations.

Caffeine is clearly addicting when consumed in sufficient quantity and is recognized by the American Psychiatric Association as such.

HISTORY

Amphetamine was first synthesized in 1887 and first used in medicine in 1927 as a stimulant and as a decongestant. Benzedrine was marketed as an inhaler in 1932. In 1937, amphetamine was first used to calm hyperactive children. It was issued to soldiers in the Second World War to counteract fatigue, elevate mood, and increase endurance. The amphetamine black market began, and students and truck drivers began using them to stay awake.

In 1949, Benzedrine inhalers were associated with overdose deaths. In the 1950s, U.S. soldiers in Korea mixed amphetamine with heroin to create the first "speedball." Amphetamines began to be prescribed for narcolepsy, chronic fatigue, and obesity. In the 1960s, widespread abuse began. Intravenous methamphetamine became a popular drug of abuse. Users were known as "speed freaks." Runs occur with methamphetamine in the same manner as they do with cocaine. The black market flourished. In the 1970s and 1980s, cocaine replaced much of the amphetamine abuse.

Recently, a new form of methamphetamine called "ice" has been encountered on the U.S. mainland. Originating in Hawaii, it is a smokable form of methamphetamine, much like crack is a smokable form of cocaine. The main difference is the fact that the effects of ice last 4 to 5 hours, whereas those of cocaine last only 20 to 30 minutes.

DRUG CULTURE NAMES

Names for amphetamines in the drug culture include:

Drug	Drug culture names	
amphetamine sulfate	bennies	whites
	peaches	copilots
dextroamphetamine	copilots	oranges
	dexies	footballs
methamphetamine	crystal	speed
	crank	quartz
	glass	ice
	meth	

Drug	Drug culture names	
dextroamphetamine + amphetamine sulfate	black beauties black birds	black mollies

ACTIONS

The actions of amphetamines, and other stimulant drugs in sufficient quantity, are virtually identical to those of cocaine. In addition, caffeine acts as a diuretic, increasing urine output.

ABSTINENCE SYNDROME

The abstinence syndrome for amphetamines and other stimulant drugs is identical to that of cocaine. The caffeine withdrawal headache is thought to be due to the vasoconstrictive effect of caffeine on blood vessels in the brain and the vasodilation that occurs when the drug is abruptly discontinued.

HEALTH CONSEQUENCES

A number of adverse health consequences arise from stimulant abuse. They are identical to those produced by cocaine.

In the last few years, abuse of Vick's nasal inhalers has been reported. To use the drugs, abusers prepare a solution by dripping a weak solution of hydrochloric acid over a wick from the inhaler to extract the stimulant, L-desoxyephedrine. The mixture is then injected into a vein to achieve a "cheap" high. The author treated one young addict who had been told about the procedure by a friend and decided to try it. He was not able to get the needle into one of the usual venous sites in the arms so he decided to try to inject the material into the femoral vein, a large vein located deep in the groin area. Unfortunately, he missed the vein and injected it into the tissues around it, resulting in death of the tissues about

½-inch deep and 3 inches in diameter. The damage had to be repaired surgically.

CONCLUSIONS

Stimulants other than cocaine include amphetamines, amphetamine cogeners, methylphenidate (Ritalin), phenylpropanolamine, and caffeine.

Amphetamines now have few medical uses. In resistant cases they are sometimes used to treat hyperactive children and narcolepsy, a condition in which people have trouble staying awake.

The amphetamine cogeners (Tenuate, Preludin, Fastin) are prescription diet pills. Ritalin is used to treat hyperactive children.

Phenylpropanolamine is an ingredient in decongestants and over-the-counter diet pills.

Caffeine, an ingredient in coffee, tea, and soft drinks, is also present in over-the-counter cold and allergy medications, diet pills, stimulants, and headache remedies.

Ice, a new form of methamphetamine, has spread from Hawaii to the U.S. mainland. It is highly addictive and its effects last much longer than those of cocaine.

The actions of amphetamines and other stimulants are qualitatively similar to those of cocaine, as are the withdrawal symptoms and health consequences.

Cannabinoids

Cannabinoids are derivatives of the Indian hemp plant, *Cannabis sativa*. The plant contains more than 60 cannabinoids, of which delta-9-tetrahydrocannabinol (THC) is the major psychoactive substance. It also contains several carcinogens.

THE CANNABINOID DRUGS

Marijuana

This is the dried flowering tops, leaves, and stems of the hemp plant, which are usually chopped up and smoked in cigarette form, called a joint, or in pipes. It can be eaten as well. Marijuana is the main cannabinoid abused in the United States. It is a particular favorite of adolescents. Marijuana looks like dried parsley with stems and/or seeds. Chopped marijuana resembles grass clippings from which the name "grass" comes. In the United States, the THC concentration of most marijuana is 1 to 2 percent. The most potent form of marijuana is known as *sinsemilla*, with a THC concentration that averages about 7 percent. The marijuana smoked today is three to four times as potent as the marijuana smoked ten years ago. Substances that are sometimes mixed with marijuana in an attempt to increase its potency include PCP, opium, formaldehyde, and Raid insect spray.

Hashish

This is the resinous extract of the hemp plant. It is obtained by boiling the parts of the plant that are covered with the resin in a solvent or by scraping the resin off. Hashish is a very potent form of cannabis, with a THC concentration of 5 to 12 percent. Hashish comes in brown or black cakes or balls, and is smoked or eaten.

Hash Oil

This is an even more potent form of cannabis, having a THC concentration of 20 to 50 percent. Hash oil is a concentrated syrupy liquid varying in color from clear to black. It is usually smoked in a water pipe (bong) to regulate the intake and cool the smoke, or is mixed with tobacco.

The active compound, THC itself, comes in soft gelatin capsules and is ingested orally.

HISTORY

Cannabis use dates back thousands of years. Marijuana was referred to in a Chinese pharmacology treatise in 2737 BC, and a reference to its use in 2000 BC was found in India. An urn containing marijuana was found in Germany dating back to 500 BC, indicating early introduction of the drug into Europe. In 1545, the Spaniards introduced the hemp plant to South America, and around 1611 early colonists in Virginia cultivated the plant for fibers from which they made cloth. Its use in medicine began in 1850, and during the latter half of the 19th century it was used to treat pain, convulsive disorders, hysteria, asthma, rheumatism, and labor pains.

In 1875, "hasheesh houses" modeled after opium dens began to appear in the United States. During prohibition, when alcohol use decreased, marijuana use increased. It was linked to a crime wave in the 1930s, and its use as a medicine was prohibited in 1937 by the Marijuana Tax Act. During the 1950s and 1960s its use spread to high school and college campuses. It was placed in Schedule I by the Controlled Substance Act of 1970, which made possession of marijuana a misdemeanor and intent to sell or transfer it a felony.

DRUG CULTURE NAMES

Drug culture names for marijuana include:

A-bomb (marijuana + heroin)	Maryjane
AMP (marijuana + formaldehyde)	M.J.
doobie	pot
grass	reefer (marijuana cigarette)
hay	roach (butt end of marijuana
hemp	cigarette)
Jane	supergrass (high potency
joint (marijuana cigarette)	marijuana, marijuana + PCP)
kiff (marijuana + tobacco)	tea

ACTIONS

The most prominent effects of marijuana are

1. *Brain*
    - an increased sense of well-being
    - euphoria
    - sense of detachment
    - feelings of relaxation and sleepiness

- short-term memory impairment
- depersonalization (a sense of strangeness and unreality about one's self)
- balance difficulty
- impaired perception, attention, and information processing
- vivid visual imagery
- impaired psychomotor function
- a keener sense of hearing
- subtle visual and auditory stimuli take on a novel character
- altered perception of time (time seems to pass more slowly)
- increased hunger, called "marijuana munchies"
- antiemetic effect (reduced nausea and vomiting)

2. *Cardiovascular*
   - increased heart rate
   - decreased blood pressure when standing up
   - marked reddening of the conjunctiva (eyes)

3. *Other*
   - decreased sweating
   - increased body temperature
   - decreased intraocular (eye) pressure
   - dry mouth and throat
   - muscle weakness
   - tremors

ABSTINENCE SYNDROME

People who suddenly stop smoking marijuana after heavy, long-term use may experience withdrawal symptoms:

- irritability, restlessness, and nervousness
- decreased appetite
- mild tremor and chills

- mildly increased body temperature
- increased REM sleep—the part of sleep associated with dreams
- marijuana craving

It is unclear if there is a postacute abstinence syndrome associated with marijuana use. Because of its mild nature, the marijuana abstinence syndrome does not require medication.

HEALTH CONSEQUENCES

Marijuana use causes concern about adverse health effects, in part because so many of its users are young. Effects include

- bronchoconstriction (airway constriction)
- pharyngitis (inflammation of the throat)
- sinusitis (inflammation of the sinuses)
- bronchitis (inflammation of the airways)
- increased risk of lung cancer
- decreased sperm count and mobility
- disruption of the menstrual cycle
- aggravation of angina pectoris (heart pain)
- suppressed immunity

Heavy, long-term marijuana smoking by adolescents is said to produce the *amotivational syndrome*, which consists of loss of energy, apathy, absence of ambition, loss of effectiveness, inability to carry out long-term plans, impaired memory, and a marked decline in school performance. Evidence does not support the notion that smoking marijuana causes permanent brain damage.

THERAPEUTIC APPLICATIONS

The substance THC does have some possible therapeutic applications, including the treatment of nausea and vomiting produced by cancer chemotherapy agents, and the treatment of increased intraocular (eye) pressure that leads to glaucoma. To date, although it has been studied, it has not been approved for these applications.

CONCLUSIONS

Marijuana produces stimulatory effects, a sense of depersonalization, altered perception of time, and hunger. It contains a number of cancer-producing agents.

Marijuana withdrawal symptoms are mild; however, heavy, long-term use of marijuana can lead to the amotivational syndrome and can cause a number of health problems. Among these, lung cancer is a theoretical consequence.

Marijuana does have some possible therapeutic applications, such as treatment of nausea produced by cancer chemotherapy and glaucoma.

27

Phencyclidine

THE PHENCYCLIDINE DRUGS

Phencyclidine (PCP) is an illegal substance appearing in the form of a white to off-white crystalline powder that is easily and inexpensively synthesized from readily available, legal chemicals. At least 60 PCP-related drugs have been developed. Phencyclidine is most commonly mixed with marijuana, tobacco, oregano, or parsley, and then smoked. It can also be snorted, taken as a pill or liquid by mouth, or injected intravenously. Phencyclidine is abused for its euphoric effects, its ability to decrease inhibition, its ability to instill feelings of power and eliminate pain, and the altered perceptions of time, space, and body image it produces.

Fortunately, PCP use has become fairly uncommon in recent years. The author has seen two noteworthy cases. One was a young man who was dragged into the emergency room, fighting all the way, by four burly policemen. His indiscretion had been to show up for church naked and in a psychotic state. It took an equal number of male orderlies to hold him down long enough to sedate him. A drug screen was positive for PCP. Nudity in public is one of the bizarre behavioral manifestations of PCP intoxication.

The most dramatic response to PCP the author has seen was in another patient brought to the emergency room by the police. He had been found in a comatose state in a local motel room.

Despite the coma, his eyes were wide open, and all of his muscles were intensely contracted to the point where he had done a considerable amount of damage to them. His CPK (an enzyme in the blood used to assess muscle damage) was 123,500. The normal range is 5 to 55. We gave him a large intravenous dose of diazepam (Valium), which normally is an excellent muscle relaxant, but it had no effect.

To prevent further muscle damage, we had to admit him to the intensive care unit (ICU) and start him on Pavulon (a drug similar to curare) to paralyze him. Because the drug also paralyzes the respiratory muscles and renders patients unable to breathe, he had to be intubated and placed on a ventilator to breathe for him. The myoglobin that had spilled out of his damaged muscles plugged up his kidneys so that he went into kidney failure and had to be placed on an artificial kidney machine. During his stay in the ICU, he developed a blood-clotting disorder and bled into one of his lungs. A pulmonary physician then had to bronchoscope him and suck the blood clots out of his lung. Despite the stormy course during his one-month stay in the ICU, he recovered enough to refuse treatment for drug addiction and returned home.

HISTORY

Phencyclidine was first manufactured in 1957 by the pharmaceutical company Parke-Davis Laboratories and entered into human studies shortly afterward. It was developed to be a less-dangerous anesthetic than the ones we had then and still have today. It worked well; however, 10 to 20 percent of the people it was administered to acted bizarrely upon awakening. They became extremely agitated and some had seizures or epileptic fits. Because of these effects, its use as a human anesthetic was discontinued in 1965. However, PCP continued to be manufactured and marketed from 1965 to 1978 as a veterinary anesthetic since it did not have these effects on animals. Its use in veterinary medicine explains many of its drug-culture names. All PCP manufactured since 1979 has been done so illegally.

The first illegal use of PCP appeared on the streets of San Francisco in 1967 in the form of a pill known as a PeaCe Pill, from which comes its name—PCP. It rapidly developed a bad reputation because it was regularly associated with "bad trips" that resulted in dangerous behavior. Because of this, it fell into disfavor, only to resurface a few years later, when smoking the drug, which allowed titration of its effects, became popular. Because it is inexpensive to manufacture, PCP is frequently misrepresented by dealers as another drug, most often as LSD, mescaline (peyote), psilocybin (mushrooms), or cocaine.

DRUG CULTURE NAMES

Drug culture names for PCP include:

angel dust	monkey dust
animal tranquilizer	PCP
crystal	PeaCe Pill
dust	rocket fuel
elephant tranquilizer	selma
embalming fluid	sherman
D.O.A. (dead on arrival)	super cools
gorilla biscuits	supergrass (PCP + marijuana)
hog	superweed
horse tranquilizer	wackey weed
krystal joint	zombie dust

ACTIONS

The typical dose of PCP produces a variety of physical and psychological effects.

1. *Physical effects*
   - loss of concentration
   - illogical speech
   - dysarthria (difficulty pronouncing words)
   - blunted response to pain
   - ataxia (a staggering gait)
   - muscle rigidity
   - grimacing and bruxism (chewing motions)
   - nystagmus (rapid, involuntary eye movements)
   - a blank stare
   - elevated temperature
   - increased pulse rate and breathing rate
   - elevated blood pressure
   - nausea and vomiting
   - flushing, lacrimation (tearing), and salivation

2. *Psychological effects*
   - unpredictable behavior
   - drunken and euphoric appearance
   - impaired perception of danger
   - delusions of invulnerability
   - altered perception of time, space, and distance
   - alternating periods of lethargy and fearful agitation
   - negative attitude or hostility
   - disorganized thoughts
   - combative and violent behavior, sudden rage
   - feelings of disassociation from one's body
   - stereotyped behavior (sucking, picking, and repetitive movements)
   - users appear unable to speak
   - catatonia (trance-like state)
   - echolalia (involuntary repetition of a word or sentence just spoken by another person)
   - socially uninhibited (obscenity or nudity in public)
   - feelings of inordinate strength (often described as feeling like they could stand in front of a locomotive and stop it with their bare hands)

- psychosis indistinguishable from paranoid schizophrenia or mania (extremely hyperactive behavior and thinking)

When used in an excess dose, the PCP user may lapse into a coma in which the eyes remain open in a fixed stare and all of the muscles in his body contract violently, producing muscle damage.

ABSTINENCE SYNDROME

Acute withdrawal signs and symptoms following cessation of PCP use include nervousness, anxiety, and depression. Uses may experience a postacute abstinence syndrome consisting of depression and loss of recent memory, which may last for months or years. The acute abstinence syndrome is not severe enough to require medication; however, the depression of the postacute abstinence syndrome may respond to antidepressant medication.

HEALTH CONSEQUENCES

- Injuries due to violence or self-destructive behavior
- Muscle damage and kidney failure
- Liver damage
- Aspiration pneumonia (breathing one's own vomitus)
- Heart failure and pulmonary edema (excess fluid in the lungs)
- Hypertensive encephalopathy (delirium produced by excessively high blood pressure)
- Seizures or epileptic fits
- Malignant hyperthermia (excessively high body temperature)
- Intracranial hemorrhage (bleeding into the skull)
- Coma, death

CONCLUSIONS

Phencyclidine was developed by the pharmaceutical industry as an anesthetic. Because of bizarre side effects, however, it never became widely used in humans, although it was used in animals for a period of years. Legal manufacture ceased in 1979, but since it is easily and inexpensively manufactured, clandestine laboratories have continued to manufacture it. Phencyclidine produces a number of psychological and physical effects among which is the feeling of superhuman strength. This often leads to injuries in the user.

Acute withdrawal symptoms are mild; however, protracted depression can be a problem.

Health consequences of PCP abuse can be severe—kidney failure, liver damage, intracranial hemorrhage, coma, and death.

28

Inhalants

The inhalants are either volatile liquid substances whose fumes are inhaled directly, or gases that are inhaled. They include solvents and aerosols, nitrites, and nitrous oxide.

THE INHALANT DRUGS

Solvents and Aerosols

Solvents and aerosols are complex compounds of distilled petroleum and natural gas. They are liquids at room temperature, but evaporate readily. Abused substances in this group include:

cements and glues	Liquid Paper
cleaning solutions	paint thinners
Freon	Scotchgard
gasoline	spot removers
lacquers	varnish
lighter fluid	varnish remover

Adolescent boys most commonly abuse solvents and aerosols recreationally because they have access to many household products and do not have access to more conventional drugs. Most adolescents inhale the substance either directly or from a solvent-soaked rag. Another method, known as *bagging*, involves placing a piece of cotton or a solvent-soaked rag in the bottom of a paper bag that is then placed over the nose and inhaled. Solvent and aerosol inhaling is known as *huffing*.

Nitrites

The nitrites include amyl nitrite and butyl nitrite. Amyl nitrite is a prescription drug used to alleviate angina (heart pain). It comes as a clear yellowish liquid in ampules that are broken, and the fumes may be inhaled. It is a favored drug in the homosexual population because it helps relax the anal sphincter, making penetration easier.

Butyl nitrite has similar properties. It comes in small bottles as room deodorizers and liquid incense. It is widely and legally sold in novelty stores, tape and record shops, drug paraphernalia stores, and by mail order. It is often used in discotheques to promote a sense of abandon. One brand is reported to bear a warning label, "Warning, if inhaled this product may produce euphoria."

A word of warning is appropriate here. If your child has taken to regularly using liquid incense in his room, it is more likely that butyl nitrite is being abused or the smell of marijuana is being covered up rather than your teenager being concerned about having a nice-smelling room.

Nitrous Oxide

Nitrous oxide is used medically as a dental anesthetic, and is known as *laughing gas*. Dentists sometimes abuse it and become addicted to it. The author knows of a dentist who strapped a tank of nitrous oxide to the back of the front seat of his car and connected it by plastic tubing to a nasal biprong so that he could drive to work and back while breathing the substance. He swore he wasn't addicted to it.

Nitrous oxide is commonly used in the food industry. Aerosol whipped-cream containers, referred to in the drug cultures as *whippits*, use it as the propellant. These containers are widely available in grocery stores and other food outlets. Adolescents obtain the nitrous oxide from the containers using a special device that is also readily available in various stores. Nitrous oxide is also available as an additive for automobile engines. Furthermore, it can readily be made in illicit laboratories.

Whippits (small metal cylinders containing nitrous oxide), balloons for inhaling the gas, and pipes for smoking it (called "buzz bombs") are sold in drug paraphernalia shops. Although drugs such as cocaine are illegal in all states, in many of them it is legal to sell drug paraphernalia.

HISTORY

Inhaling substances for their euphoric and intoxicating effects has a long history. Thousands of years ago, people inhaled vapors from burning spices and herbs, particularly as part of religious ceremonies.

Solvents and Aerosols

Gasoline inhaling began to be reported as a recreational activity in the 1950s. In the 1960s, glue sniffing became a national concern when several deaths were reported. In the 1970s, solvents and aerosols came into widespread use as inhalants. In the 1980s, inhaling substances such as Liquid Paper, used to correct typewriter errors, and Scotchgard, used to stainproof upholstery, became popular. Deaths from abuse of both of these substances have occurred. Local and state governments now prohibit minors from purchasing certain substances, particularly plastic model glues.

Nitrites

Amyl nitrite was discovered in 1857 and abuse of it became popular in the 1970s as enhancers of sexual experience, especially among male homosexuals. At that time, it was an over-the-counter medication used to treat angina. It is supplied in small glass vials that are broken open to inhale the vapors. Because of the sound the breaking makes, amyl nitrite became known in the drug culture as *poppers*. When it was made a prescription drug in 1980, butyl nitrite, because it is easily obtained, replaced it as a drug of abuse. The medical use of amyl nitrite, which is still available by prescription, has been replaced by nitroglycerin.

Nitrous Oxide

Nitrous oxide was used for recreation long before it was used medically. Discovered in the 1700s, nitrous oxide was most commonly abused by students and physicians. Inhalant parties were popular in the 1800s. A detailed description of nitrous oxide's analgesic (pain relief) and anesthetic properties was published in the 1800s. Despite this, its potential for abuse and dependence was not recognized until the latter part of the 1960s. Since then, the nonmedical use of nitrous oxide has been on the rise.

DRUG CULTURE NAMES

Drug culture names for various inhalants include:

Drug	Drug culture names	
amyl nitrite	amies	poppers
	amys	snappers
	pearls	
butyl nitrite	banaple gas	rush

Drug	Drug culture names	
butyl nitrite (*cont.*)	joc aroma	Satan's scent
	kick	thrust
	locker popper	toilet water
	locker room	
nitrous oxide	laughing gas	whippits

ACTIONS

Solvents and Aerosols

Solvents and aerosols cause:

- excitement, irritability, and restlessness
- a lowering of inhibitions
- changes in perception
- uncoordination
- confusion and disorientation
- impaired judgment
- sedation

Nitrites

The nitrites produce:

- dilation of peripheral blood vessels
- decreased return of blood to the heart
- relaxation of the rectal sphincter
- euphoria

Nitrous Oxide

Nitrous oxide produces:

- relaxation and sedation

- reduced pain
- mild heart muscle depression
- intoxication
- euphoria

ABSTINENCE SYNDROME

An abstinence syndrome consisting of hallucinations, abdominal cramps, chills, and delirium tremens has been reported with heavy chronic abuse of solvents. If an abstinence syndrome does occur, however, it happens rarely. An abstinence syndrome for nitrites and nitrous oxide has not been reported.

HEALTH CONSEQUENCES

Solvents and Aerosols

These substances are extremely toxic when inhaled. They can cause

1. *Neurological*
   - ataxia or an unsteady gait
   - paralysis of peripheral and cranial nerves
   - headache
   - delirium
   - delusions and hallucinations
   - syncope (passing out)
   - seizures
   - respiratory depression
   - permanent brain damage
   - coma

2. *Cardiovascular*
   - anemia
   - cardiac arrhythmias and cardiac arrest

3. *Gastrointestinal*
   - loss of appetite and weight loss
   - nausea and vomiting
   - gastritis
   - liver damage and jaundice (yellow discoloration of the skin)
4. *Kidneys*
   - kidney damage
5. *Musculoskeletal*
   - myopathy (muscle damage)
6. *Skin*
   - rash around mouth and nose or on the hands
7. *Other*
   - lead poisoning (from leaded gasolines)

Deaths from solvents and aerosols occur for several reasons. Death from suffocation occurs when a user loses consciousness and falls on a cloth containing one of the solvents. Suffocation from a plastic bag placed over the head to concentrate the vapors also occurs.

Aerosol abuse can cause death from laryngospasm or freezing of the airways. Freon can cause death by blocking the uptake of oxygen across the membranes of the lungs. The most dramatic health hazard of abusing solvents and aerosols is the *sudden sniffing death (SSD) syndrome*, which results from the effect of the substances on the heart, causing cardiac arrest.

Nitrites

Adverse health consequences of the nitrites include

- headache
- methemoglobinemia (decreased capacity of the blood to carry oxygen)
- irritation of the eyes

- irritation of the airways
- crusty lesions around the mouth and nose
- burns
- hemolysis (destruction of red blood cells)
- suppression of the immune system
- speeding up the progression of AIDS

Nitrous Oxide

Adverse health consequences of nitrous oxide result primarily from the fact that it inactivates vitamin B_{12}.

Physical effects
- distal limb weakness
- mild loss of vibratory sensation
- paresthesias (altered sense of pain and touch in the limbs)
- decreased ankle and knee reflexes
- gait abnormalities
- bladder and bowel dysfunction

Psychological effects
- depression
- loss of recent memory
- confusion and delirium
- paranoid delusions
- visual hallucinations

Nitrous oxide can also depress the activity of heart muscle, which can have disastrous consequences in individuals with heart trouble.

Deaths have also occurred from nitrous oxide abuse. There has been at least one death from ruptured airways as a result of trying to inhale the gas directly from the tank without a pressure-reduction valve.

Deaths have also occurred when sufficient oxygen to support life was not mixed with the nitrous oxide. A young medical student recently died from nitrous oxide abuse. He was on call one night in the hospital and decided he would get "high." He somehow managed to get small tanks of nitrous oxide and oxygen from the anesthesiology service, along with the appropriate device for reducing the pressure and mixing the gases. Unfortunately for him, the mask he got was one that strapped on. After inhaling the mixture for awhile, the oxygen ran out, and he suffocated. He was found the next morning in one of the small departmental libraries, still sitting in the chair with the mask on.

CONCLUSIONS

Inhalants are either volatile liquid substances whose fumes are inhaled, or gases that are inhaled directly. They include solvents, aerosols, nitrites, and nitrous oxide.

Adolescent boys most commonly abuse solvents and aerosols because these substances are inexpensive and are readily available. Adverse health consequences from abuse of these drugs include effects on most organ systems of the body. Permanent brain damage is an unfortunate sequela. Deaths from cardiac arrest sometimes occur.

Amyl nitrite is a prescription drug once used to treat angina. Butyl nitrite is found in room deodorizers and liquid incense. Adverse health consequences from abuse of these drugs include red blood cell destruction, suppression of the immune system, and speeding up of the process of AIDS.

Nitrous oxide (laughing gas) is widely used as an anesthetic in dentists' offices. Adverse health consequences of its abuse include distal limb weakness, bladder and bowel dysfunction, depression, confusion, delusions, and hallucinations.

29

Anabolic Steroids

Anabolic steroids are used primarily in an attempt to increase muscle mass and athletic performance. They are more accurately called anabolic–androgenic steroids because they produce an *anabolic effect*, which is protein synthesis for building muscle, and an *androgenic effect*, or masculinization, due to their testosterone-like properties.

THE ANABOLIC STEROID DRUGS

All anabolic steroids in use today are derivatives of the male sex hormone, testosterone. They are legally manufactured for a few legitimate medical reasons, but probably 80 percent of them are diverted to the black market for unsupervised use. Anabolic steroids come in tablet and injectable forms. Some of the more common ones are:

Generic name	Trade name
Oral forms	
ethylestrenol	Maxibolin, Orabolin
fluoxymesterone	Halotestin, Android-F
methandrostenolone	Dianabol

Generic name	Trade name
methyltestosterone	Android, Metandren, Oreton, Testred, Vigorex, Virilon
norethandrolone	Nilevar
oxandrolone	Anavar
oxymetholone	Anadrol-50, Adroyd

Injectable forms

nandrolone decanoate	Deca-Durabolin
nandrolone phenpropionate	Durabolin
testosterone cypionate	DEPO-Testosterone
testosterone enanthate	Delatestryl
testosterone propionate	Oreton

Injectable steroids are absorbed directly into the bloodstream, thereby avoiding the first-pass effect of the liver. The first-pass effect refers to the fact that ingested drugs must pass from the intestines through the liver in order to reach the bloodstream. The liver metabolizes a major part of the oral dose in this process. In addition, by avoiding the first-pass effect, injectable steroids are less toxic to the liver than the oral ones.

Anabolic Steroid Users

It has been estimated that more than 80 percent of athletes involved in body building, national and international weightlifting, power-lifting, and field events such as shotput and discus throw use steroids. One-half of professional football linemen and linebackers are thought to use the drugs. A number of female athletes, especially those involved in body building and power-lifting, are steroid users. Estimates of steroid use among college athletes have ranged from 5 to 20 percent.

What about adolescents? A recent study of steroid use in a large suburban high school revealed that 4.4 percent of students used anabolic steroids (6.5 percent males, 2.5 percent females). Athletes had a higher rate of use (5.5 percent) than nonathletes. Use was highest among wrestlers (13.3 percent) and football players (12.2 percent) and lowest for track athletes (4.0 percent) and swimmers (5.0 percent). Students reported obtaining the drugs from coaches (23 percent), physicians (33 percent), friends (43 percent), and other sources (24 percent). One-third of high school anabolic steroid users reported beginning use prior to age 16.

Adolescent boys who do not compete in sports sometimes use anabolic steroids in an attempt to make themselves look more attractive to the opposite sex.

Method of Use

To maximize the anabolic effect, while minimizing the health risks and likelihood of being detected by drug screens, a regimen called *pyramiding* is often used by athletes. For example, an individual might use the first 3 weeks of a 12-week regimen before a competition to inject himself or herself weekly with 200 mg of testosterone cypionate and ingest 10 mg of one of the oral forms daily. During the next three weeks, the dose of the injected drug might be increased to 400 mg and the dose of the oral drug to 15 mg. For weeks 7 and 8, the weekly dose of the testosterone cypionate might be raised to 600 mg, the oral drug to 20 mg, and a second oral drug added, a process known as *stacking*. During weeks 9 and 10 the dose of the injected drug is reduced to 200 mg per week. The oral doses remain the same. During week 11, the first oral drug is discontinued, as is the injectable one. During week 12, the second oral drug is discontinued. To avoid being caught by a urine drug screen, no drugs are used the final week before the competition. Athletes have been known to use 10 to 40 times the normal daily dose.

Denial

Denial plays a major role in steroid abuse:

- Users do not believe that they are causing harm to anyone—a "victimless crime."
- Athletes feel that they must use them if they want to compete seriously with others whom they believe are using the drugs.
- They deny that anabolic steroid use has significant adverse health consequences. They make statements like, "Every drug, even aspirin, has side effects."
- They condemn those who criticize the use of anabolic steroids. "People who are against steroid use are not athletes. They just don't understand."
- They appeal to higher loyalties, sort of a code of commitment to the sport. Those competing at the international level may view anabolic steroid use as a patriotic act.

HISTORY

The search for a superman formula has a long history. In the late 1800s, the famous neurologist, Brown-Seguard, administered to himself a testicular extract containing testosterone. Testosterone itself was synthesized in the laboratory in 1935, and used in an attempt to help chronically ill people replace lost muscle mass. Steroids were reportedly given to German troops during the Second World War to increase their aggressiveness.

The anabolic steroids were recognized as having potential for use among athletes in the early 1950s, and Russian weightlifters began to use analogues of testosterone in 1954. The practice spread to the United States in the late 1950s.

In 1973, the American Academy of Pediatrics stated that anabolic steroid use by adolescents was detrimental to their health. In 1976, the International Amateur Athletic Federation banned their use, and in 1977 the American College of Sports Medicine officially opposed use of the drugs. During the 1983 Pan American Games, several athletes were disqualified when anabolic steroids were detected by urine drug screens, and dozens more withdrew from the games for fear of detection. The National Collegiate Athletic Association (NCAA), in 1986, began drug-testing college football players in selected games, and the California Legislature placed anabolic steroids under controls and imposed penalties for trafficking. Ben Johnson, the Olympic sprinter who set a world record in the 100-meter dash in 1988, was disqualified after testing positive for steroids.

The United States Congress in the Anabolic Steroid Act of 1990, classed these drugs in Schedule III.

ACTIONS

Individuals who use steroids do so in the belief that these drugs:

- increase body mass
- increase muscle mass
- increase strength
- increase aggressiveness
- improve times in running events
- reduce recovery time after a workout
- increase intensity at which weight training can be done
- increase the length of workout periods
- promote rapid healing of injuries
- allow them to keep up with their opponents
- give them the winning edge
- make them look more attractive to the opposite sex

Whether anabolic steroids actually do all of these things is debatable. Research has shown that they do not improve performance in aerobic athletic events, such as the sprint races. They do seem to increase strength in weightlifters who have undergone intensive training before beginning anabolic steroid use.

ABSTINENCE SYNDROME

The anabolic-steroid abstinence syndrome consists primarily of depression, which may be severe. Suicides have been reported. Another withdrawal symptom is viewed as being the opposite of anorexia nervosa. Those suffering from anorexia nervosa see themselves as overweight despite being merely skin and bones. Anabolic steroid abusers see themselves as being undermuscled despite the fact that they may appear to others as having a tremendous physique. The 10 to 25 pounds they lose on cessation of anabolic steroid use takes on an exaggerated importance, a phenomenon which has been termed *megarexia*.

HEALTH CONSEQUENCES

A number of adverse effects can result from anabolic steroid abuse. Many of them are irreversible.

1. *Liver*
   - Liver damage that is indicated by elevated liver enzymes in the blood
   - Cholestatic jaundice (yellow skin color resulting from obstruction of bile flow)
   - Peliosis hepatis (venous lakes in the liver, prone to rupture)
2. *Endocrine*
   - Acne (both sexes) due to proliferation of sebaceous glands
   - Altered glucose metabolism
   - Suppressed testosterone levels in men
   - Reduced sperm count with infertility

- Feminization of males: development of female-like breasts (gynecomastia) and shrunken testicles
- Masculinizing effects in women: this includes hoarsening of the voice, hirsutism (development of male-like body hair patterns), enlargement of the clitoris, decrease in breast size, menstrual irregularities, and male pattern baldness
- Premature sexual development in children

3. *Skeleton*
   - Premature closure of epiphyseal growth plates, which limits a person's height

4. *Cardiovascular*
   - Increased risk of cardiovascular disease, due to decreased levels of HDL-cholesterol and increased levels of LDL-cholesterol
   - Hypertension (high blood pressure)
   - Elevated triglyceride levels
   - Fluid retention

5. *Behavioral*
   - Irritability
   - Aggressive behavior, termed "'roid rage"
   - Euphoria
   - Decreased fatigue
   - Changes in libido
   - Mood swings
   - Hallucinations
   - Manic-like symptoms (severe hyperactivity of thoughts and actions)
   - Paranoid delusions (feelings that others are out to get you)

The aggressive behavior produced by anabolic steroids can be a significant problem. The author was told of one young athlete who, in a 'roid rage, walked along the street bashing parked cars with a crowbar. When confronted by the police, he attacked them with the crowbar. Despite being shot repeatedly, he kept coming after them, before finally falling dead at their feet.

CONCLUSIONS

Anabolic steroids are derivatives of the male sex hormone, testosterone. They produce protein synthesis for muscle building and masculinization, even in women. Abuse rates among professional athletes is said to be high. These drugs are also abused by some college and high school athletes and especially by body builders.

Anabolic steroids are abused because users believe that these drugs increase muscle mass and strength, increase aggressiveness, promote rapid healing of injuries, and give them "the winning edge."

Withdrawal consists mainly of depression, which can be severe. Adverse health consequences from abuse of these drugs involve the liver, endocrine system, skeleton, and cardiovascular system. Behavioral problems include aggressiveness, mood swings, hyperactivity, and paranoid delusions.

30

Hallucinogens

THE HALLUCINOGENIC DRUGS

The hallucinogenic drugs are favorites of adolescents. They include a variety of substances whose *psychedelic* effects range all the way from simple visual distortions to frank hallucinations. The hallucinogens include the following drugs.

LSD (Lysergic Acid Diethylamide)

LSD, usually known as "acid" in the drug culture, is derived from a substance found in a parasitic fungus that grows on rye and other grains. It is a white, odorless material that is usually mixed with colored material when sold illegally. It is manufactured as a capsule, tablet, or liquid, as well as impregnated on blotter paper or in thin gelatin squares. It can be taken orally or licked off blotter paper. In addition, gelatin and liquid can be put into the eyes. It is an extremely potent drug so that only a very small amount has to be used. It is a popular drug of adolescents.

Psilocybin

Psilocybin is the active hallucinogenic ingredient in *Psilocybe mexicana* mushrooms and a few other species. Adolescents identify this particular mushroom because it tends to grow in cow dung and because it has an unusual expansion of the trunk. The mushrooms are chewed or swallowed.

Mescaline

Mescaline is the active hallucinogenic ingredient in the peyote cactus, which is found in northern Mexico and Texas. Mescaline comes as hard brown discs, tablets, and capsules. The discs are chewed, swallowed, or smoked. The tablets and capsules are taken orally.

MDMA (Ecstasy)

Ecstasy is a derivative of methamphetamine. MDEA (Eve), a derivative of amphetamine, is similar to ecstasy. The drugs come as white powders, tablets, and capsules. They are taken orally.

Nutmeg

Nutmeg, a common cooking spice, is the dried seed of *Myristica fragrans*, an evergreen tree indigenous to east India. It is closely related to mescaline. Nutmeg is usually mixed in tea, hot chocolate, or orange juice and then drunk.

Morning Glory Seeds

Morning glory seeds are first pulverized and soaked in water, then the water is strained and drunk. Morning glory seeds are readily available legally, and can even be ordered from mail-order catalog companies.

Mappine (Bufotenine)

Mappine is extracted from the skin and glandular secretions of the toad *Bufo marinus*. Its psychoactive effects can be experienced by grinding up the dried skin and smoking it or simply licking the toad. It is also found in the mushroom *Amanita mappa* and the shrub *Piptadinia peregrina*.

HISTORY

LSD

LSD was synthesized in the laboratory in 1938 during experimentation with ergot fungus. Its accidental ingestion in 1943 led to the discovery of its psychedelic properties. From 1949 to 1954, LSD was widely studied. The U.S. Army tested it for use as a brainwashing agent and as a way of making prisoners talk more readily. Psychiatrists believed that its effects mimicked schizophrenia and used it in an attempt to better understand mental illness. It was used widely by psychiatrists as an adjunct to psychotherapy.

Until 1960, illegal use of LSD was restricted to a small number of intellectuals. Its illegal use on a broad scale began in the United States in 1962. Dr. Timothy Leary, an instructor at Harvard University, recommended that everyone should "turn on, tune in, and drop out." Chronic users of LSD are known as "acid heads."

LSD seems to be making a comeback. The newest fad, "rave" parties, consists of several hundred young people meeting at a designated site, such as an abandoned warehouse, and partying nonstop for several days. LSD is the principal drug used at these gatherings.

Psilocybin

Ritual use of mushrooms by Mexican and Central American cultures dates back to 1500 BC. The mushrooms were considered sacred and were called "flesh of the gods." In 1958, psilocybin, the active ingredient, was identified as the psychoactive substance in mushrooms.

Mescaline

Mescaline has been used in religious rites since the earliest recorded time, and, although an illegal drug, its use is allowed by the Native American Church. The active ingredient of the peyote cactus, mescaline was isolated in 1897, and its chemical structure was determined in 1918.

MDMA (Ecstasy)

MDMA was developed by the pharmaceutical industry and used legally by psychiatrists in the 1970s to facilitate psychotherapy. Since 1983, it has been a popular drug of abuse among adolescents and young adults. In 1985, the Drug Enforcement Administration placed MDMA in Schedule I. Despite this, it continues to be manufactured illegally. A small group of psychiatrists still lobby for its legal use in psychotherapy because they believe it to be helpful. MDEA (Eve) is also manufactured illegally. It appeared in the drug culture in 1985 and was placed in Schedule I in 1987.

Mappine

Mappine was used by the Vikings, as well as natives of Siberia and the Caribbean. Its use by adolescents has been relatively recent.

DRUG CULTURE NAMES

The hallucinogenic drugs are known by a variety of names in the drug culture.

Drug	Drug culture names	
LSD	acid	L
	big D	lysergide
	blotter acid	microdots
	blue heaven	pellets
	cubes	sugar cubes
	deeda	wedges
	dots	window panes
psilocybin	magic mushrooms	shrooms
	mushrooms	silly putty
	sacred mushrooms	
mescaline	bad seeds	mesc
	beans	mescal
	big chief	moon
	buttons	p
	cactus	peyote
MDMA	Adam	M & M
	ectasy	X
	lovedrug	XTC
MDEA	Eve	
morning glory seeds	Bindweeds	Heavenly Blues
	Blue stars	Pearly Gates
	Flying Saucers	Wedding Bells
mappine	yopo	cohoba

ACTIONS

LSD

The effects produced by LSD depend on the quantity of the drug used and the user's psychological and emotional state, as well as the setting in which the drug is used. It causes:

- Alterations in perception. Colors seem brighter and objects appear to have rainbows around them
- Distortion of shape and size of objects
- Boundaries of objects seem to shift and dissolve
- Synesthesia (seeing music as a series of colors and shapes)
- Time seems to pass very slowly
- Hallucinations
- Pupillary dilation
- Increased body temperature
- Increased heart rate
- Increased blood pressure
- Muscle weakness
- Tremor

Psilocybin

The effects produced by psilocybin are similar to those of LSD. In addition, in large doses, numbness in the tongue, lips, or mouth may occur.

Mescaline

The effects produced by mescaline are also similar to those of LSD. However, it is considerably less potent.

MDMA (Ecstasy)

The effects produced by MDMA depend on the dose. In low doses it produces the desired effects. In high doses it produces stimulant effects.

Low dose	High dose
euphoria	increased heart rate
enhanced self awareness	elevated blood pressure
visual distortions	increased breathing rate
	increased temperature
	mydriasis (dilated pupils)
	tremor

MDEA (Eve) causes effects similar to those of MDMA, but milder.

Morning Glory Seeds

Morning glory seeds produce effects similar to those of LSD. However, the active ingredient is about one-tenth as potent as LSD.

Mappine

Mappine produces altered perceptions of time and space, and can produce hallucinations.

ABSTINENCE SYNDROME

Use of hallucinogenic drugs is not associated with an abstinence syndrome.

HEALTH CONSEQUENCES

LSD

The main disturbing effect of LSD use is the *flashback*, a reexperiencing of the effects of the drug weeks or even months after last using it. There is no evidence that even long-term, high-dose use of LSD causes permanent damage to the body or brain.

Death or injuries occasionally occur when, under the influence of the drug, the user decides, for example, that he can fly and leaps from a tall building. Deaths and injuries have also occurred when users experienced flashbacks at inappropriate times, such as when driving an automobile.

Psilocybin

Like LSD, there is no evidence that long-term, high-dose psilocybin causes permanent damage to the body or brain, other than the accidental deaths and injuries discussed above.

Mescaline

In low doses, the health effects of mescaline are similar to those of LSD. In high doses, however, it causes:

- fever
- headache
- drop in blood pressure
- decreased heart and lung function

Long-term health consequences are not known to occur from mescaline use.

MDMA (Ecstasy)

Animal studies suggest that MDMA may destroy the presynaptic nerve cell endings in the brain that contain serotonin in their storage vesicles. Deaths due to cardiac arrest have been associated with its use. Deaths have also occurred from MDEA use.

Nutmeg

The use of nutmeg causes:

- vomiting
- excessive thirst
- constipation
- difficulty urinating

Long-term health consequences are not known to occur.

Morning Glory Seeds

The use of morning glory seeds can cause:

- nausea, vomiting, and diarrhea
- intense headache
- drowsiness
- chills
- impaired vision
- decreased blood pressure
- shock

Long-term health consequences are not known to occur from morning glory seed use.

Mappine

Effects produced by mappine include:

- seizures
- high blood pressure
- cardiac arrhythmias (irregular heartrate)
- coma
- death from cardiac arrest

The skin of a single toad contains enough mappine to be fatal.

CONCLUSIONS

The hallucinogenic group of drugs are also known as psyche-delics. They include LSD, psilocybin (mushrooms), MDMA (ec-stasy), mescaline, nutmeg, morning glory seeds, and mappine from toads. They produce effects ranging from visual distortions to frank hallucinations. The most disturbing aspect of their use is a phenomenon known as flashbacks, a reexperiencing of the ef-fects of the drug weeks to months after last using it.

The use of hallucinogens is not associated with withdrawal symptoms.

Long-term adverse health consequences do not occur from hallucinogen abuse; however, deaths from suicide and injuries while under the influence have occurred.

Epilogue

This book began by saying that there are 15 questions to which parents and teachers should know the answers. The following is a brief discussion of these questions and their answers.

1. *What are drugs of abuse?* Drugs of abuse are substances that alter the way people feel, and which are capable of producing addiction.

2. *How do drugs of abuse differ from other drugs?* Drugs of abuse possess a number of characteristics that other drugs do not. In addition to altering the way people feel and producing addiction, the drugs themselves reinforce drug use, often cause withdrawal symptoms, and produce drug craving. They do all this by altering the functioning of certain chemicals in the brain known as neurotransmitters.

3. *Is alcoholism truly a disease?* Evidence indicates that alcoholism is a disease and that it possesses biological, psychological, and social characteristics. For many individuals, the tendency to develop the disease is transmitted genetically.

4. *Why do adolescents abuse drugs?* Adolescents abuse drugs for a number of reasons; however, the reason given most commonly is that drugs make them feel good and they do not believe that drugs cause them any harm.

341

5. *Can drug abuse be prevented?* Evidence clearly indicates that drug-abuse prevention efforts do work. Prevention, however, requires perseverance, consistency, and a planned program. Parents, teachers, and counselors can play important roles.

6. *How can I tell if my child is abusing drugs?* The key to the diagnosis of chemical dependence is the assessment, which consists of medical, psychological, and social evaluations. Urine drug screening is an important part of the medical evaluation.

7. *What can I do if my child is abusing drugs?* If it is determined that a child is chemically dependent, several options are open to the parents—tough love, confrontation, or court order to a treatment facility. If it is determined that the child is not chemically dependent but merely using drugs experimentally, a contract between parents and child should be signed in which the adolescent agrees to stop the drug use and to voluntarily enter a treatment program if he continues to use drugs. If he does continue to use but refuses to enter a treatment program, tough love, confrontation, or court order can be instituted.

8. *What does treatment entail?* Treatment of chemically dependent adolescents most commonly takes the form of inpatient treatment, outpatient treatment, or a combination of the two. It consists primarily of education, insight development, and behavior modification. Group and individual therapy, stress management, and support groups such as Alcoholics Anonymous are important components.

9. *Do young women have special issues?* Women often have a number of issues that need to be addressed, such as childcare, dysfunctional relationships, and sexuality. In addition, if pregnant, they may have concerns about what drinking and using has done to their unborn child.

10. *What help is available to the rest of the family?* The effects of drug abuse on the user's family can be profound. Help is available, however, usually in the form of family or codependency programs at local treatment facilities. In addition, support groups such as Al-Anon and Alateen are also usually available. As families recover, they gradually take on the characteristics of a healthy family.

11. *What happens when my child comes home from treatment?* Support groups and aftercare attendance are vital parts of recovery. The recovery process generally proceeds through a number of successive stages until a maintenance stage is attained. A number of prescription and over-the-counter medications can be hazardous to this process. With both adolescent and other family members working their programs, family recovery can proceed in an orderly fashion.

12. *What if he uses drugs again?* Relapse is an ever-present concern. Relapse, like recovery, is a process. Taking a drink or using a drug is the last stage of this process. A number of factors, such as dishonesty, stress, and overconfidence, can lead to relapse. Should relapse occur, a number of steps should be taken by the adolescent to get back into his recovery program. If he is not willing to take these steps and continues to drink or use, tough love, confrontation, or court order can be reinstituted.

13. *Does drug abuse cause mental problems?* Drug abuse, per se, does not cause mental illness; however, symptoms resulting from intoxication, overdose, and withdrawal can mimic virtually any mental disorder. Additionally, drug abuse sometimes complicates the lives of people who have true mental illness.

14. *How are drug abuse and AIDS related?* AIDS has been reported in all fifty states and in at least one hundred countries worldwide. Infected individuals remain in an asymptomatic carrier state for a number of years before developing the full-blown disease. During this stage they can transmit the virus to others. AIDS is ultimately fatal. The most common mode of transmission is sexual contact, both heterosexual and homosexual. The second most common mode of transmission is intravenous drug use. A significant proportion of sexual transmission cases occurs between infected drug abusers and their heterosexual partners.

15. *Do I have problems of my own which I need to work on?* Many drug-abusing adolescents are members of dysfunctional families. Having grown up in an alcoholic family is a common cause of this dysfunction. Alcoholic families tend to develop a set of dysfunc-

tional rules to help them deal with the stress of their situation. In addition, individual members tend to assume certain dysfunctional roles. People growing up in alcoholic families (Adult Children Of Alcoholics) tend to carry dysfunctional characteristics into adulthood. If you are an ACOA, you may need counseling and/or you may need to join an ACOA support group.

Appendixes

Appendix A

Sources of Help
and Information

For information on where to find treatment for alcohol and other drug problems, the best place to look is in the telephone book's Yellow Pages under "Alcoholism Information" or "Drug Abuse and Addiction Information."

Useful 1-800 Numbers

1-800-729-6686
National Clearinghouse for Alcohol and Drug Information
Monday through Friday, 9:00 a.m.–7:00 p.m.

1-800-622-HELP
National Institute on Drug Abuse Information and Referral Line
Monday through Friday, 9:00 a.m.–3:00 a.m.

1-800-554-KIDS
The National Federation of Parents for Drug-Free Youth
Monday through Friday, 9:00 a.m.–5:00 p.m.

1-800-622-2255
National Council on Alcoholism
7 days a week, 24 hours a day

1-800-241-9746
Parent's Resource Institute for Drug Education (PRIDE)
Monday through Friday, 8:30 a.m.–5:00 p.m. (recorded service other times)

1-800-COCAINE
Cocaine Helpline
Monday through Friday, 9:00 a.m.–3:00 a.m.
Saturday and Sunday, 12:00 p.m.–3:00 a.m.

Private Organizations, Civic Groups, and Religious Organizations

Adult Children of Alcoholics
 (ACOA)
P.O. Box 3216
Torrance, CA 90505
(213) 534-1815

Al-Anon Family Groups
P.O. Box 862
Midtown Station
New York, NY 10018
(212) 302-7240
1(800) 344-2666

Alcoholics Anonymous (AA)
15 E. 26th Street, Rm 1810
New York, NY 10010
(212) 683-3900

American Counsel for Drug
 Education
204 Monroe Street, Suite 110
Rockville, MD 20850
(301) 294-0600
1(800) 488-DRUG

American Society for Addiction
 Medicine (ASAM)
5225 Wisconsin Ave NW, #409
Washington, DC 20015-2016
(202) 244-8948

The Chemical People/WQED
1 Allegheny Square
Suite 720
Pittsburgh, PA 15212
(412) 391-0900

Cocaine Anonymous (CA)
3740 Overland Avenue
Suite G
Los Angeles, CA 90034
(213) 559-5833
1(800) 347-8998

CoAnon Family Groups
P.O. Box 64742-66
Los Angeles, CA 90064
(213) 859-2206

Families Anonymous, Inc.
P.O. Box 528
Van Nuys, CA 91408
(818) 989-7841

Institute on Black Chemical
  Abuse
2616 Nicollet Avenue
Minneapolis, MN 55408
(612) 871-7878

Just Say No Foundation
1777 North California Blvd.
Room 210
Walnut Creek, CA 94596
(415) 939-6666
1(800) 258-2766

Mothers Against Drunk Driving
  (MADD)
511 E. John Carpenter Freeway
Suite 700
Irving, TX 75062
(214) 744-6233

Nar-Anon Family Groups
P.O. Box 2562
Palos Verdes Peninsula, CA 90274
(213) 547-5800

Narcotics Anonymous (NA)
P.O. Box 9999
Van Nuys, CA 91409
(818) 780-3951

National Families in Action
2296 Henderson Mill Road
Suite 204
Atlanta, GA 30345
(404) 934-6364

National Federation of Parents for
  Drug-Free Youth
9551 Big Bend
St. Louis, MO 63122
(314) 968-1322

National Parents Resource
  Institute for Drug Education
  (PRIDE)
The Hurt Building
50 Hurt Plaza, Suite 210
Atlanta, GA 30303
(404) 577-4500

National Asian Pacific American
  Families Against Drug Abuse
6303 Friendship Court
Bethesda, MD 20817
(301) 530-0945

National Association for Children
  of Alcoholics (NACoA)
31582 Coast Highway
Suite B
South Laguna, CA 92677
(714) 499-3889

National Association of State
  Alcohol and Drug Abuse
  Directors (NASADAD)
444 N. Capitol Street, NW
Suite 642
Washington, DC 20001
(202) 783-6868

National Black Alcoholism and
  Addictions Council (NBAC)
1629 K Street, NW
Suite 802
Washington, DC 20006
(202) 296-2696

National Coalition of Hispanic
Health and Human Services
Organizations (COSSMHO)
1030 15th Street, NW
Suite 1053
Washington, DC 20005
(202) 371-2100

National Council on Alcoholism
and Drug Dependence
(NCADD)
12 W 21st Street
New York, NY 10010
(212) 206-6770

National Prevention Network
444 North Capitol Street, NW
Suite 642
Washington, DC 20001
(202) 783-6868

Quest International
537 Jones Road
P.O. Box 566
Granville, OH 43023
(614) 587-2800

Women for Sobriety
P.O. Box 618
Quakertown, PA 18951
(215) 536-8026

Appendix B

Recommended Reading for Children

Elementary School Children

A Little More About Alcohol, 1984. Alcohol Research Information Service, 1120 East Oakland Avenue, Lansing, MI 48906. $0.75. A cartoon character explains facts about alcohol and its effects on the body.

Alcohol: What It Is, What It Does, by Judith S. Seixas, 1977. Greenwillow Books, 105 Madison Avenue, New York, NY 10016. An easy-to-read illustrated primer on the use and abuse of alcohol.

An Elephant in the Living Room: The Children's Book, by Marion H. Hyppo and Jill M. Hastings, 1984. CompCare Publications, P.O. Box 27777, Minneapolis, MN 55427. An illustrated workbook designed to help children from alcoholic homes understand that alcoholism is a disease and that they are not alone in coping with its effects.

Buzzy's Rebound, by William Cosby and Jim Willoughby, 1986. National Clearinghouse for Alcohol and Drug Information, P.O. Box 2345, Rockville, MD 20852. An 18-page "Fat Albert" comic book that describes the pressure on a new kid in town to drink.

Kids and Alcohol: Get High On Life, by Jamie Rattray et al., 1984. Health Communications, Inc. 1721 Blount Road, Suite 1, Pompano Beach, FL 33069. A workbook designed to help children (ages 11–14) make important decisions in their lives and feel good about themselves.

Kootch Talks About Alcoholism, by Mary Kay Schwandt, 1984. Serenity Work, 1455 North University Drive, Fargo, ND 58102. A 40-page coloring book in which Kootch the worm helps young children understand alcoholism and alcoholics.

The Sad Story of Mary Wanna or How Marijuana Harms You, by Peggy Mann, illustrated by Naomi Lind, 1988. Woodmere Press, P.O. Box 20190, Cathedral Finance Station, New York, NY 10025. A 40-page activity book for children in grades 1–4 that contains pictures of the damage that marijuana does to the body.

Whiskers Says No to Drugs, 1987. Weekly Reader Skills Books, Field Publications, 245 Long Hill Road, Middletown, CT 06457. This book contains stories and follow-up activities for students in grades 2 and 3 to provide information and form attitudes before they face peer pressure to experiment.

Secondary School Children

Chew or Snuff Is Real Bad Stuff. National Cancer Institute, U.S. Department of Health and Human Services Building 31, Room 10A24, Bethesda, MD 20892. This 8-page pamphlet describes the hazards of using smokeless tobacco.

Christy's Chance, 1987. Network Publications, P.O. Box 1830, Santa Cruz, CA 95061-1830. A story geared to younger teens that allows the reader to make a nonuse decision about marijuana.

Different Like Me: A Book for Teens Who Worry About Their Parents' Use of Alcohol/Drugs, 1987. Johnson Institute, 7151 Metro Boulevard, Minneapolis, MN 55435. This 110-page book provides support and information for teens who are concerned, confused, scared, and angry because their parents abuse alcohol and other drugs.

Don't Lose a Friend to Drugs, 1986. National Crime Prevention Council, 1700 K Street, N.W., 2nd Floor, Washington, DC 20006. This brochure offers practical advice to teenagers on how to say "no" to drugs, how to help a friend who uses drugs, and how to initiate community efforts to prevent drug use.

Source: A Parent's Guide to Prevention: Growing Up Drug Free. U.S. Department of Education, Washington, DC, 1990.

Appendix C

Recommended Videos
for Parents, Teachers,
and Counselors

A Gift for Life: Helping Your Children Stay Alcohol and Drug Free, 1989. American Council on Drug Education, 204 Monroe Street, Suite 110, Rockville, MD 20850.

Drug-Free Kids: A Parent's Guide, 1986. Scott Newman Center, 6255 Sunset Blvd., Suite 1906, Los Angeles, CA 90028.

Say NO! to Drugs: A Parent's Guide to Teaching Your Kids How To Grow Up Without Drugs and Alcohol, 1986. PRIDE, The Hurt Building, 50 Hurt Plaza, Suite 210, Atlanta, GA 30303. Order No. F008S.

Source: A Parent's Guide to Prevention: Growing Up Drug Free. U.S. Department of Education, Washington, DC, 1990.

Glossary

Abstinence Living without the use of psychoactive substances.

Abstinence Syndrome The unpleasant signs and symptoms following discontinuation of a drug to which the user has become addicted.

Acid Head A habitual heavy user of LSD.

ACOA (Adult Children of Alcoholics) A support program aiding adults with problems resulting from having had alcoholic parents.

Addict A person who is presently, or has been in the past, addicted to one or more drugs, including alcohol.

Aftercare A structured recovery program that follows treatment. It may be a few months to two years in length.

Al-Anon A support organization for family and close friends of alcoholics.

Alateen A support organization for the teenage children of alcoholics.

Alcoholic A person with the disease of alcoholism; an addict whose addiction is to alcohol.

Alcoholics Anonymous (AA) The prototype, and largest, of the support groups.

Alcoholism A chronic, progressive illness characterized by significant impairment that is directly associated with persistent and excessive consumption of alcohol. Impairment may involve medical, psychological, or social dysfunction.

Amotivational Syndrome A state of passive withdrawal from usual work, school, and recreational activities due to chronic, heavy marijuana use.

Bad Trip A frightening reaction after the use of a hallucinogenic drug.

357

Balloons   Drugs are sometimes packaged for sale in balloons.

Basing   Using freebase cocaine.

Bender   Being on a drug spree.

Big Book   The book, *Alcoholics Anonymous,* written by active members of Alcoholics Anonymous describing the behavior and characteristics of alcoholics.

Big Man   The person who supplies a pusher with drugs.

Blackout   A temporary loss of memory caused by alcohol or other drug intoxication.

Blood Alcohol Level (BAL) or Concentration (BAC)   Concentration of alcohol in the blood.

Bomb   A large-size marijuana cigarette; also, high-quality heroin which has been diluted very little.

Bombed Out   Feeling the effects of a drug.

Bong   A water pipe used to smoke marijuana. The smoke bubbles through the water and eliminates some of the harshness.

Book, The   The *Physicians' Desk Reference;* also called "the Bible."

Boost   To shoplift. A common way for an adolescent to obtain money to buy drugs.

Booting   Attempting to prolong the initial effects of a heroin injection by injecting a small amount, then withdrawing blood back into the syringe and repeating the process.

Bottoming Out   When a person has reached a level of emotional, spiritual, and physical harm, due to drug abuse, that he or she can no longer tolerate.

Brick   A pressed block of marijuana, opium, or morphine. In the case of marijuana, it weighs one pound.

Bummer   A frightening reaction after using a drug.

Burn   Cheating or being cheated in drug deals.

Burned Out   Refers to a chronic drug user who is weary of the hassle of obtaining drugs, or heavy marijuana smokers who become dull and apathetic and withdraw from their usual activities.

Buzz   Feeling the effects of a drug, usually alcohol or marijuana.

Buzz Bomb   Pipe for smoking nitrous oxide.

Candy   Drugs.

Candy Man   A person who sells drugs.

Cent   In drug language a cent refers to a dollar, a nickel is $5, a dime is $10.

Chemical Dependence   A chronic, progressive illness characterized by significant impairment that is directly associated with persistent and excessive use of alcohol or another drug. Impairment may involve medical, psychological, or social dysfunction.

Chipping   Using drugs irregularly and infrequently.

Clean   Not using or possessing drugs.

Coast   To experience the drowsy, somnolent effects of heroin.

Cocaine Anonymous (CA)   Support group similar to AA but for cocaine addicts.

Codependent   One who lets another person's behavior affect him or her and who is obsessed with controlling that person's behavior.

Coke Head   A heavy user of cocaine.

Coke Whore   A person who sells sex to get cocaine.

Cold Turkey   Quitting using a drug without the benefit of medication.

Come Down   Returning to a normal state after drug effects have worn off. For heroin addicts this state signals the beginning of withdrawal symptoms.

Cook   Heating heroin powder with water until it dissolves and is ready for injection.

Cop   The act of purchasing a drug.

Crack   Freebased form of cocaine HCl; so named because of the crackling sound it makes when it is smoked.

Crack House   A house whose main purpose is the selling and smoking of crack cocaine.

Crash   Suddenly falling asleep after the heavy use of stimulants or to rapidly return to a normal state when the drug effects have worn off.

Cross Addiction   A recovering addict who has been dependent on one drug is a potential setup for addiction to any drug.

Cross Tolerance   The development of tolerance to drugs in the same class as the abused drug.

Crossing the Wall   Passing from the use/abuse stage into the addiction stage. Thought to involve central nervous system neurotransmitter derangement.

Deal   To sell illicit drugs.

Dealer   A person who sells drugs.

Delirium Tremens   Severe form of alcohol withdrawal; occurs in Stage 4 of the alcohol abstinence syndrome.

Denial   Symptom of chemical dependence characterized by the subconscious lack of recognition of a problem even in the face of significant adverse consequences, and despite the fact that the problem is evident to others.

Dependence   See *Drug Addict*.

Designer Drug   Substance resulting from minor changes in the molecular structure of a parent drug to avoid prosecution for the manufacture of a scheduled drug. The psychoactive properties are retained.

Detoxification   The process by which a drug-addicted person returns to normal physical and mental functioning; this may be accomplished by the abrupt end of drug use (cold turkey), or by gradual discontinuation of the drug under medical supervision.

Dime   In drug language, a dime refers to $10.

Dirty   Having drugs in one's possession (opposite of clean).

Disulfiram (Antabuse)   Medication to help support recovery from alcoholism.

Dollar   In drug language, a dollar refers to $100.

Dope   Narcotic drugs.

Dried Out   Detoxified from a drug.

Drug   A substance that exerts a mood-altering effect on the central nervous system and which has the potential to produce addiction; includes alcohol.

Drug Addict   A person with the disease of chemical dependence, resulting from drug use other than alcohol.

Druggies   People who frequently experiment with a wide variety of drugs; also, high school or college youth who use drugs regularly.

Dry Drunk   Attitudes and behaviors of the abstinent alcoholic or drug addict that seem identical to attitudes and behaviors seen during periods of active drinking or drug use.

Dual Diagnosis   A condition in which a person has a true psychiatric disorder and chemical dependence.

Eight Ball   Approximately three grams of cocaine.

Enabler   An individual who provides the means, or opportunity, for the alcoholic or drug addict to continue psychoactive drug use.

Factory   A secret place where drugs are diluted, packaged, or prepared for sale.

Fix   The injecting of heroin or the heroin itself (also applies to using any drug intravenously).

Flashback   The recurrence of a previous drug-induced experience which occurs despite the absence of that drug.

Flashing   A term applied to sniffing glue.

Floating   Being under the effects of a drug.

Freak Out   A bad, panicky reaction to a drug.

Freebase   Smokable form of cocaine.

Front   To sell drugs to another person on credit.

Fruit Salad   A game, usually played by teenagers, in which one pill is swallowed from each bottle in a medicine cabinet.

Garbage Head   A person who will use any drug available to get high.

Get Off   To experience the effects of a drug; also, to take a heroin injection.

Geographic Cure   Moving to another location (city, state) in an attempt to "cure" one's addiction by the move alone.

Grower   A person who grows marijuana.

Halfway House   A structured transitional living situation between inpatient treatment and returning home.

Hallucination   A visual, auditory, olfactory, or tactile perception that does not exist outside of one's mind.

Hallucinosis   Visual hallucinations occurring with a relatively clear sensorium.

Head Shop   Shops that sell drug paraphernalia.

Higher Power   The "God as we understood him" of Alcoholics Anonymous.

Hit   To use a drug, particularly heroin or marijuana.

Hooked   Addicted to a drug.

Huffing   The act of inhaling the fumes of solvents or aerosols.

Hypnotic   A drug that induces sleep.

Intervention   A procedure designed to speed up the occurrence of a crisis situation to get the addict into treatment earlier than normally would occur.

Junk   Drugs, particularly heroin.

Junkie   A heroin addict.

Kick   To break a drug addiction, as in "kicking the habit."

Knockout Drops ("Mickey Finn")   A mixture of alcohol and chloral hydrate.

Lid   A measurement of weight used for marijuana; ranging from ¾ to 1 ounce.

Loaded   To be heavily intoxicated, whether from alcohol or another drug.

Loss of Control   Inability of addicts to stop alcohol or drug use once it is initiated; for example, ending up drunk when the intent was only to have a few drinks.

Minor Tranquilizers   Benzodiazepines used for sedation.

Monkey on My Back   A person's drug dependence.

Mood-Altering Drug (MAD)   A drug that makes a person feel different; a psychoactive substance.

Naltrexone (Trexan)   Medication to help support recovery from opioid addiction.

Narc   A narcotics police officer.

Narcotic   Term used to designate drugs with morphine-like actions. Comes from the word *narcosis*.

Narcotics Anonymous (NA)   Similar to AA, but designed for narcotic addicts.

Needle Habit   Some addicts, often referred to as "needle freaks," are not particular about what drug they inject but get their thrills simply from the act of injecting.

Nickel   In drug language, a nickel refers to $5.

Nickel Bag   A package, usually of marijuana or heroin, which is worth $5.

Nod   To feel the initial effects of a heroin injection (drowsiness and peacefulness) probably so called because the head nods forward.

O.D.   Overdose.

Opioid   A term used to designate all drugs (natural, semisynthetic, synthetic, agonist–antagonist) with morphine-like actions.

Paraphernalia   The equipment needed to inject heroin, smoke pot, free-base cocaine, or otherwise get high on a drug.

Partial Recovery   Low-quality sobriety resulting from failing to progress in recovery.

Physical Dependence   Addiction to a drug which is characterized by an abstinence (withdrawal) syndrome.

Pill Head   A person who frequently uses amphetamines and barbiturates or is addicted to prescription drugs.

Popping   To take a pill; also, the subcutaneous injection of heroin.

Postacute Abstinence Syndrome   Characterized by continued lesser withdrawal symptoms weeks to months past acute withdrawal.

Pot Head   A heavy user of marijuana.

Psychedelic Drugs   Drugs that induce altered states of perception, thoughts, and feelings that are not experienced otherwise except in dreams or at times of religious experiences. Hallucinogenic drugs.

Psychological Dependence   Addiction to a drug which is characterized by the absence of an abstinence (withdrawal) syndrome.

Pusher   A dealer who sells drugs directly to an addict; a person who is one step below the wholesaler in the drug distribution system.

Pyramiding   Successively adding one anabolic steroid after another until a peak is reached, then deleting one after another in preparation for an athletic event.

Recovery   A process in which the medical, psychological, and social damage caused by chemical dependence is healed. A life-long process.

Relapse   A process leading back to drinking or using. The act itself.

Residential Treatment   A form of treatment that is longer and less intense than inpatient treatment; therapeutic communities and half-way houses are forms of residential treatment.

Rig   Apparatus for injecting heroin or smoking pot.

Roach   A marijuana cigarette that has burned down too far to be held with the fingers.

Roach Clip   An instrument (pin, tweezers) used to hold a roach.

Rock Cocaine   Freebase form of cocaine produced by combining cocaine hydrochloride with baking soda, and then heating. So named because this form resembles small rocks.

Run   A period of heavy and prolonged use of a particular drug, usually referring to amphetamines or cocaine.

Rush   The initial euphoric effects occurring after a heroin or amphetamine injection.

Score   To buy a drug.

Script   A prescription for a drug; an abbreviation of the word prescription.

Script Doc   A physician who deliberately over-prescribes or misprescribes psychoactive substances for profit, or who is so easily duped that he gains a reputation for gullibility.

Sedative   A drug that relaxes and calms.

Sedative-Hypnotic   A drug that relaxes and calms but also induces sleep, depending on the dose.

Sinsemilla   A potent type of marijuana.

Set   The physiological and psychological state of a person before he or she uses a drug.

Setting   The conditions and circumstances surrounding a drug user when he or she uses the drug.

Shooting Gallery   A location where addicts inject heroin.

Shoot Up   To inject a drug, particularly heroin.

Sick   To experience the beginning of withdrawal symptoms.

Slip   A brief, short-lived relapse followed by an immediate return to abstinence.

Snow Lights   Flickering bright lights at the periphery of the visual fields that are seen after cocaine use.

Sober   A term reserved for alcoholics who work a program of recovery that includes the twelve steps of AA and emphasizes spiritual values, positive thinking, and a productive lifestyle.

Speed Freak   A heavy user of amphetamines.

Spoon   A measurement of heroin (1/16 of an ounce), or cocaine (1/4 of a teaspoon).

Stacking   Using several anabolic steroids at the same time.

Stash   A cache of hidden drugs.

Stoned   Being high on a drug.

Straight   A person who doesn't use drugs; a square; also a term for a regular cigarette.

Strung Out   An addict who has a severe addiction; or an addict's physical appearance because of a severe addiction.

Support Group   A group of people recovering from some form of drug addiction who agree to assist each other in recovery.

Target Syndrome   Successive rings of involvement (community activities, leisure activities, church, friends, peers, distant family, nuclear family) are peeled away until only the center of the target, the addict, is left.

Telescoping   The phenomenon of addiction developing more rapidly in adolescents than in adults.

Therapeutic Community   A form of residential treatment in which a minimum of professional staff is used; treatment may be confrontational.

Tight   A person who is intoxicated by alcohol or other drugs.

Toke   To smoke a marijuana cigarette; the term refers to both smoking the whole cigarette and just taking a puff.

Toke Pipes   Pipes used to smoke marijuana.

Toke Up   To light a marijuana cigarette.

Tolerance   The necessity to use, over a period of time, larger and larger doses of a drug to get high.

Toot   To snort or sniff cocaine.

Tough Love   Allowing the addict to suffer the consequences of his or her own behavior; an ultimate path to help.

Tranquilizer   See *Sedative*.

Trip   The act of using a hallucinogen, particularly LSD; or the effects of its ingestion.

Turn On   To use a drug or encourage another to do so; to feel the effects of a drug.

User   A person who uses drugs.

Wasted   To lose consciousness from drug intoxication.

Whippit   Whipped cream dispenser containing nitrous oxide as the propellant.

Wiped Out   Acute drug intoxication.

Wired   A person who is feeling the high effects of amphetamines. The term also applies to a heroin addict.

Withdrawal Syndrome   See *Abstinence Syndrome*.

Works   The apparatus for injecting narcotics, particularly heroin.

Zonked   Acutely intoxicated by a drug.

References

Chapter 1

*Bartimole, C. R. and J. E. Bartimole. *Teenage Alcoholism and Substance Abuse: Courses, Consequences, and Cures*. Frederick Fell Publishers, Hollywood, Florida, 1987.

*Beacher, G. M. and A. S. Friedman. *Youth Drug Abuse*. Lexington Books, Lexington, Massachusetts, 1979.

Farrow, J. A. Adolescent Chemical Dependency. *Adolescent Medicine*, 74(5):1265–1274, 1990.

Henderson, D. C. and S. C. Anderson. Adolescents and Chemical Dependency. *Social Work in Health Care*, 14(1):1989.

Hsu, L. K. G. and M. Hersen (Eds.). *Recent Developments in Adolescent Psychiatry*. Wiley, New York, 1989.

Milhorn, H. T., Jr. Adolescents and Drugs: Part I. *Mississippi State Medical Association Recovering Physicians Newsletter*, August, 1991.

Milhorn, H. T., Jr. Adolescents and Drugs: Part II. *Mississippi State Medical Association Recovering Physicians Newsletter*, April, 1992.

Stimmel, B. (Ed.). *Alcohol and Substance Abuse in Adolescents*. Haworth, New York, 1985.

Ungerleider, J. T. and N. J. Siegel. The Drug Abusing Adolescent: Clinical Issues. *Psychiatric Clinics of North America*, 13(3):435–442, 1990.

An asterisk (*) denotes recommended reading for parents, teachers, and counselors.

367

Chapter 2

Bratter, T. E. and G. G. Foster (Eds.). *Alcoholism and Substance Abuse*. The Free Press, New York, 1985.

Cohen, S. *The Substance Abuse Problems: Volume 1*. Haworth Press, New York, 1981.

Cohen, S. *The Substance Abuse Problems: Volume 2*. Haworth Press, New York, 1985.

Liepman, M. R., R. C. Anderson, and J. V. Fisher (Ed.). *Family Medicine Curriculum Guide to Substance Abuse*, Society of Teachers of Family Medicine, Kansas City, Missouri, 1984.

Schuckit, M. A. *Drug and Alcohol Abuse*. Plenum Press, New York, 1990.

Wilford, B. B. (Ed.). *Drug Abuse: A Guide for Primary Care Physicians*. American Medical Association, Chicago, 1981.

Chapter 3

Giannini, A. J. and N. S. Miller. Drug Abuse: A Biopsychiatric Model. *American Family Physician*, **40**:173–182, 1989.

Meltzer, H. Y. *Psychopharmacology*. Raven Press, New York, 1987.

Milhorn, H. T., Jr. Nicotine Dependence. *American Family Physician*, **39**:214–224, 1989.

Milhorn, H. T., Jr. Pharmacological Management of Acute Abstinence Syndromes. *American Family Physician*, **45**:231–239, 1992.

Milhorn, H. T., Jr. Understanding Chemical Dependence. *Journal of the Mississippi State Medical Association*, April, 1992, pp. 123–128.

Chapter 4

Blum, K. E., P. Noble, P. J. Sheridan, et al. Allelic Association of Human Dopamine D_2 Receptor Gene in Alcoholism. *Journal of the American Medical Association*, **263**:2055–2060, 1990.

Cloninger, C. R. Neurogenic Adaptive Mechanisms in Alcoholism. *Science*, **236**:410–416, 1987.

Goodwin, D. W. Alcoholism and Heredity. *Archives of General Psychiatry*. **36**:57–61, 1979.

Jellinek, E. M. *The Disease Concept of Alcoholism*. Hillhouse, New Haven, Connecticut, 1960.

Morrison, M. A. and Q. T. Smith. Psychiatric Issues of Adolescent Chemical Dependence. *Insight*, **3**:3–10, 1987.

Milhorn, H. T., Jr. The Diagnosis of Alcoholism. *American Family Physician*, **37**:175–183, 1988.

Schuckit, M. A. Genetics and the Risk of Alcoholism. *Journal of the American Medical Association*, **254**:2614–2617, 1988.

Talbott, G. D. Alcoholism and Other Drug Addictions: A Primary Disease Entity. *Journal of the Medical Association of Georgia*, 1986, pp. 490–494.

Chapter 5

*Heaslip, J., D. Van Dyke, D. Hogenson, and L. Vedders. *Young People and Drugs: Evaluation and Treatment*. Hazelden, Center City, Minnesota, 1989.

Johnston, L. D., P. M. O'Malley, and J. G. Bachman. *Drug Use by High School Seniors—Class of 1986*. U.S. Department of Health and Human Services, Rockville, Maryland, 1987.

*Krumpski, A. M. *Inside the Adolescent Alcoholic*. Hazelden, Center City, Minnesota, 1982.

Mackenzie, R. G. and E. A. Jacobs. Recognizing the Adolescent Drug Abuser. *Adolescent Medicine*, **14**:225–235, 1987.

Oetting, E. R. and F. Beauvais. Adolescent Drug Use: Findings of National and Local Surveys. *Journal of Consulting and Clinical Psychology*, **58**(4):385–394, 1990.

Chapter 6

*Isralowitz, R. and M. Singer. *Adolescent Substance Abuse: A Guide to Prevention and Treatment*. The Haworth Press, New York, 1983.

Milhorn, H. T., Jr. *Chemical Dependence: Diagnosis, Treatment, and Prevention*. Springer-Verlag, New York, 1990.

Schonberg, S. K. (Ed.). *Substance Abuse: A Guide for Professionals*. American Academy of Pediatrics, Elk Grove Village, Illinois, 1988.

Team Up for Drug Prevention with America's Young Athletes. Drug Enforcement Administration, Demand Reduction Section, Washington, D.C.

Wodarski, J. S. Adolescent Substance Abuse: Practice Implications. *Adolescence*, **25**(99):667–688, 1990.

Chapter 7

Andre, P. *Drug Addiction. Learn About It Before Your Kids Do!* Health Communications, Inc. Pompano Beach, Florida, 1987.

A Parent's Guide to Prevention. Growing Up Drug Free. U.S. Department of Education, Washington, D.C., 1990.

*Barun, K. and P. Bashe. *How to Keep the Children You Love Off Drugs*. The Atlantic Monthly Press, New York, 1988.

Drug-Free Kids: A Parent's Guide. Scott Newman Center, Los Angeles, 1986.

*Office for Substance Abuse Prevention. *10 Steps to Help Your Child Say "No"*. U.S. Department of Health and Human Services, Rockville, Maryland, 1991.

*Office for Substance Abuse Prevention. *What You Can Do About Drug Use in America*. U.S. Department of Health and Human Services. Rockville, Maryland, 1991.

*Wilmes, D. J. *Parenting for Prevention*. Johnson Institute Books, Minneapolis, 1988.

Young Children and Drugs: What Parents Can Do. The Wisconsin Clearing House, Madison, Wisconsin, 1987.

Zarek, D., J. D. Hawkins, and P. D. Rogers. Risk Factors for Adolescent Substance Abuse. Implications for Pediatric Practice. *Pediatric Clinics of North America*, **34**(2):481–493, 1987.

Chapter 8

Doing Drug Education. The Role of the School Teacher. National Institute on Drug Abuse. Rockville, Maryland, 1980.

Mississippi Substance Abuse Prevention Curriculum. Mississippi State Department of Education, Jackson, Mississippi, 1987.

*Tobias, J. *Kids and Drugs: A Handbook for Parents and Professionals*, PANDAA Press, Annandale, Virginia, 1987.

What Works: Schools Without Drugs. U.S. Department of Education. National Clearing House for Alcohol and Drug Information. Rockville, Maryland, 1989.

Chapter 9

Anglin, T. M. Interviewing Guidelines for the Clinical Evaluation of Adolescent Substance Abuse. *Pediatric Clinics of North America*, **4**:381–399, 1987.

Bernadt, N. W. and C. Taylor. Comparison of Questionnaire and Laboratory Tests in the Detection of Alcoholism. *Lancet*, **1**:325–327, 1982.

Gold, M. and C. A. Dackis. Role of the Laboratory in Suspected Drug Abuse. *Journal of Clinical Psychiatry*, **47**:17–23, 1986.

Kulberg, A. Substance Abuse: Clinical Identification and Management. *Pediatric Toxicology*, **33**:325–361, 1986.

Mullen, J. and H. S. Bracha. Toxicology Screening: How to Assure Accurate Results. *Postgraduate Medicine*, **84**:141–148, 1988.

Sanders, J. M., Jr. Identifying Substance Abuse in Adolescents. *Postgraduate Medicine*, **84**:123–136, 1988.

Chapter 10

Evans, D. G. *Kids, Drugs, and the Law.* Hazelden, Center City, Minnesota, 1985.

Griswold-Ezekoye, S., K. L. Kimpfer, and W. J. Bukoski. *Childhood and Chemical Abuse: Prevention and Intervention.* Haworth Press, New York, 1986.

*Hodgson, H. *A Parent's Survival Guide: How to Cope When Your Kid Is Using Drugs.* Harper/Hazelden, New York, 1986.

VanCleave, S., W. Byrd, and K. Revell. *Counseling for Substance Abuse and Addiction,* Word Book, Waco, Texas, 1987.

Chapter 11

Beschner, G. M. and A. S. Friedman. Treatment of Adolescent Drug Abusers. *International Journal of the Addictions,* **20**:971–993, 1985.

Henry, P. B. (Ed.). *Practical Approaches in Treating Adolescent Chemical Dependency: A Guide to Clinical Assessment and Intervention.* The Haworth Press, New York, 1989.

Jaffe, S. L. *Step Workbook for Adolescent Chemical Dependency Recovery: A Guide to the First Five Steps.* American Psychiatric Press, Washington, D.C., 1990.

Roos, S. *A Young Person's Guide to the 12 Steps.* Hazelden, Center City, Minnesota, 1992.

*Sassatelli, J. *Breaking Away: Saying Good-bye to Alcohol/Drugs.* Johnson Institute, Minneapolis, 1989.

Weger, C. D. and R. J. Diehl. *The Counselor's Guide to Confidentiality.* Program Information Associates, Honolulu, 1987.

Wheeler, K. and J. Malinquiest. Treatment Approaches in Adolescent Chemical Dependence. *Pediatric Clinics of North America,* **34**:437–447, 1987.

Chapter 12

Blume, S. Women and Alcohol. In *Alcoholism and Substance Abuse: Strategies for Clinical Intervention.* (T. E. Bratter and G. G. Forrest, Eds.). Free Press, New York, 1985, pp. 623–638.

Chesnoff, I., Jr. Drug Use in Pregnancy. Parameter of Risk. *Pediatric Clinics of North America,* **35**:1403–1412, 1988.

Holiday, A. and B. Bush. Women and Alcohol Abuse. In *Alcoholism: A Guide for the Primary Care Physician.* (H. N. Barnes, M. D. Aronson, and T. L. Delbanco, Eds.). Springer-Verlag, New York, 1987, pp. 176–180.

Martin, J. N., R. W. Martin, L. W. Hess, S. W. McColgin, J. F. McCall, and J. C. Morrison. Pregnancy-Associated Substance Abuse and Addiction: Current

Concepts and Management. *Journal of the Mississippi State Medical Association*, **29**:369–374, 1988.

Reed, B. G. Drug Misuse and Dependency in Women: The Meaning and Implications of Being Considered a Special Population. *International Journal of Addictions*, **20**:13–62, 1985.

Silverman, S. Interaction of Drug-Abusing Mother, Fetus, Types of Drugs Examined in Numerous Studies. *Journal of the American Medical Association*, **26**:1689–1690, 1989.

Smith, C. G. and R. H. Asch. Drug Abuse and Reproduction. *Fertility and Sterility*, **48**:355–373, 1987.

Chapter 13

Al-Anon Family Groups. Al-Anon Family Groups Headquarters, New York, 1987.

Al-Anon's Twelve Steps and Twelve Traditions. Al-Anon Family Groups Headquarters, New York, 1988.

Bagley, C. *Today's Promise: A Treatment Program for Families*. Laurel Wood Center, Meridian, Mississippi, 1992.

*Beattie, M. *Codependent No More*. Hazelden Press, Center City, Minnesota, 1987.

Cermak, T. L. *Diagnosing and Treating Codependence*. Johnson Institute Books, Minneapolis, 1986.

Coombs, R. H. *The Family Context of Adolescent Drug Abuse*. Haworth Press, New York, 1988.

Curran, D. *Traits of A Healthy Family*. Winston Press, Minneapolis, 1983.

Mulry, J. T. Codependency: A Family Addiction. *American Family Physician*, **35**:215–219, 1987.

Talbott, G. D. and E. B. Benson. Impaired Physicians: The dilemma of identification. *Postgraduate Medicine*, **68**:56–64, 1980.

Van Cleave, S., W. Byrd, and Revell, K. *Counseling for Substance Abuse and Addiction*. Word Books, Waco, Texas, 1987.

Chapter 14

Alcoholics Anonymous. Alcoholics Anonymous World Services, Inc., New York, 1976.

Fuller, R. K. and Williford, W. D. Life-table of Abstinence in a Study Evaluating the Efficacy of Disulfiram. *Alcoholism*, **4**:298–301, 1980.

Gonzales, J. P. and R. N. Brogden. Naltrexone: A Review of Its Pharmacodynamic Properties and Therapeutic Efficacy in the Management of Opioid Dependence. *Drugs*, **35**:192–213, 1988.

Gorski, T. T. *Passages Through Recovery*. Harper & Row/Hazelden, San Francisco, 1989.

*Hodgson, H. W. *Parents Recover Too: When Your Child Comes Home from Treatment*. Hazelden, Center City, Minnesota, 1988.

Taylor, J. R., J. E. Helzer, and N. Robins. Moderate Drinking in Ex-alcoholics: Recent Studies. *Journal of Studies on Alcohol*, 47:115–121, 1986.

Talbott, G. D. Alcoholism and Other Drug Addictions: A Primary Disease Entity. *Journal of the Medical Associates of Georgia*, 1986, pp. 490–494.

The Twelve Steps and Twelve Traditions. Alcoholics Anonymous World Services, Inc., New York, 1976.

Chapter 15

Gorski, T. T. and M. Miller. *Staying Sober: A Guide for Relapse Prevention*. Independence Press, Independence, Missouri, 1986.

Milhorn, H. T., Jr. Relapse: The Mind–Body Connection. *The Counselor*, National Association of Alcohol and Drug Abuse Counselors, September/October, 1991. pp. 16–18.

Peterson, R. L. Toward an Era of Relapse Prevention in Chemical Dependency: What Can Dentistry Do to Help? *Journal of the Michigan Dental Association*, 7(10):547–54, 1989.

Chapter 16

Diagnostic and Statistical Manual of Mental Disorders, Third Edition Revised (DSM-III-R). American Psychiatric Association, Washington, D.C., 1987.

Evans, K. and J. M. Sullivan. *Dual Diagnosis: Counseling the Mentally Ill Substance Abuser*. The Gilford Press, New York, 1990.

Morrison, M. A. and Q. T. Smith. Psychiatric Issues of Adolescent Chemical Dependence. *Insight*, 3:3–10, 1982.

Wilford, B. B. (Ed.). *Review Course Syllabus*. American Society of Addiction Medicine, New York, 1990.

Chapter 17

Amin, N. M. Acquired Immunodeficiency Syndrome, Part I: Epidemiology, History, and Etiology. *Family Practice Recertification*, 9:36–58, 1987.

Battjes, R. G., C. G. Leukefeld, R. W. Pickens, and H. W. Haverkos. The Acquired Immunodeficiency Syndrome and Intravenous Drug Abuse. *Bulletin on Narcotics*, 40:21–34, 1988.

Kaplin, M. H. The AIDS Epidemic and the Drug Substance Abuse Patient. *Journal of Substance Abuse Treatment*, **4**:127–136, 1987.

Sulima, J. P. *What Every Substance Abuse Counselor Should Know About AIDS*, Mannisses Communications Group, Washington, D.C., 1987.

Chapter 18

Friel, J. and L. Friel. *Adult Children: The Secrets of Dysfunctional Families*. Health Communications, Inc., Deerfield Beach, Florida, 1988.

Milhorn, H. T., Jr. The Alcoholic Family: Part 1. *Mississippi State Medical Association Recovering Physicians Newsletter*, December, 1990.

Milhorn, H. T., Jr. The Alcoholic Family: Part 2. *Mississippi State Medical Association Recovering Physicians Newsletter*, March, 1991.

*Wegscheider-Cruse, S. *Another Chance*. Science and Behavioral Books, Palo Alto, California, 1981.

*Woititz, J. G. *Adult Children of Alcoholics*. Health Communication, Inc., Deerfield Beach, Florida, 1983.

Chapter 19

Cohen, S. *The Chemical Brain*. Care Institute, Irvine, California, 1988.

Gilman, A. G., L. S. Goodman, T. W. Rall, and F. Murad (Eds.). *The Pharmacological Basis of Therapeutics*. Macmillan, New York, 1991.

Katzung, B. G. (Ed.). *Basic and Clinical Pharmacology*, Appleton and Lange, Norwalk, Connecticut, 1987.

Shlafer, M. and E. Marieb. *The Nurse, Pharmacology, and Drug Therapy*. Addison-Wesley, Redwood City, California, 1989.

Chapter 20

Barnes, H. N., M. D. Aronson, and T. L. Delbanco (Eds.). *Alcoholism: A Guide for the Primary Care Physician*. Springer-Verlag, New York, 1987.

Hodges, D. L. Effects of Alcohol on Bone, Muscle, and Nerve. *American Family Physician*, **34**:149–156, 1986.

Vellinek, E. M. *The Disease Concept of Alcoholism*. Hillhouse, New Haven, Connecticut, 1960.

Landers, D. F. Alcohol Withdrawal Syndrome. *American Family Physician*, **27**:114–118, 1983.

Packard, R. C. The Neurological Consequences of Alcoholism. *American Family Physician*, **14**:111–115, 1976.

Spickard, A. and B. R. Thompson. *Dying for a Drink: What You Should Know About Alcoholism*. Word Books, Waco, Texas, 1985.

Chapter 21

Bertino, J. S., Jr. and M. D. Reed. Barbiturate and Nonbarbiturate Sedative-Hypnotic Intoxication in Children. *Pediatric Clinics of North America*, **33**:703–722, 1986.

Laux, G. and D. A. Puryear. Benzodiazepines: Misuse, Abuse, and Dependency. *American Family Physician*, **30**:139–147, 1984.

Milhorn, H. T., Jr. *Chemical Dependence: Diagnosis, Treatment, and Prevention*. Springer-Verlag, New York, 1990.

Smith, D. E. and D. R. Wesson. Benzodiazepine Withdrawal Syndromes. *Journal of Psychoactive Drugs*, **15**:85–95, 1983.

Chapter 22

Milhorn, H. T., Jr. *Chemical Dependence: Diagnosis, Treatment, and Prevention*. Springer-Verlag, New York, 1990.

Seymour, R. D., D. Smith, D. Inaba, and M. Londsy. *The New Drugs: Look-alike, Drugs of Deception, and Designer Drugs*. Hazelden, Center City, Minnesota, 1989.

Chapter 23

Dackis, C. A. and M. S. Gold. Psychopharmacology of Cocaine. *Psychiatric Annals*, **18**:528–530, 1988.

Kleber, H. D. Cocaine Abuse: Historical, Epidemiological, and Psychological Perspectives. *Journal of Clinical Psychiatry*, **49**:3–6, 1988.

Vereby, K. and M. S. Gold. From Coca Leaves to Crack: The Effects of Dose and Routes of Administration on Abuse Liability. *Psychiatric Annals*, **18**:513–520, 1988.

Wyatt, R. J., F. Karourn, R. Suddeth, and A. Hitri. The Role of Dopamine in Cocaine Use and Abuse. *Psychiatric Annals*, **18**:531–534, 1988.

Chapter 24

Clementz, G. L. and J. D. Dailey. Psychotropic Effects of Caffeine. *American Family Physician*, **37**:167–172, 1988.

Dilsaner, S. C., N. A. Vololatro, and N. E. Alessi. Complications of Phenylpropanolamine. *American Family Physician*, **39**:201–206, 1989.

Dupont, R. L. *Getting Tough on Gateway Drugs*. American Psychiatric Publishing, Washington, D.C., 1984.

Halle, A. B., R. Kessler, and M. Alvarez. Drug Abuse with Vicks Nasal Inhaler. *Southern Medical Journal*, **78**:761–762, 1985.

Jackson, J. G. Hazards of Smokable Methamphetamine. *New England Journal of Medicine*, **321**:907, 1989.

Chapter 25

Cheeseboro, M. J. Passive Smoking. *American Family Physician*, **37**:212–218, 1988.

Cummings, K. M., C. R. Jaen, and G. Giovino. Circumstances Surrounding Relapse in a Group of Recent Smokers. *Prevention Medicine*, **14**:195–202, 1985.

McCusker, K. Landmarks of Tobacco Use in the United States. *Chest (Supplement)*, **93**:34–36, 1988.

Silvis, G. L. and C. L. Perry. Understanding and Deterring Tobacco Use among Adolescents. *Pediatric Clinics of North America*, **34**:363–378, 1987.

U.S. Public Health Service. *Report of the Surgeon General: Nicotine Addiction*. U.S. Department of Health and Human Services. Rockville, Maryland, 1988.

Chapter 26

*Dupont, R. L. *Getting Tough on Gateway Drugs*. American Psychiatric Publishing, Washington, D.C., 1984.

Milhorn, H. T., Jr. *Chemical Dependence: Diagnosis, Treatment, and Prevention*. Springer-Verlag, New York, 1990.

Schwartz, R. H. and D. E. Smith. Hallucinogenic Mushrooms. *Clinical Pediatrics*, **27**:70–73, 1988.

Chapter 27

Milhorn, H. T., Jr. Diagnosis and Management of Phencyclidine Intoxication. *American Family Physician*, **43**:1293–1302, 1991.

Milhorn, H. T., Jr. *Chemical Dependence: Diagnosis, Treatment, and Prevention.* Springer-Verlag, New York, 1990.

Young, T., G. W. Lawson, and C. B. Gacono. Clinical Aspects of Phencyclidine (PCP). *The International Journal of the Addictions*, **22**:1–15, 1987.

Chapter 28

Cohen, S. Volatile Nitrites. *Journal of the American Medical Association*, **241**:2077–2078, 1979.

Fortenberry, D. J. Gasoline sniffing. *American Journal of Medicine*, **8**:36–51, 1985.

Gillman, M. A. Nitrous Oxide, an Opioid Addictive Agent. *The American Journal of Medicine*, **81**:97–102, 1986.

King, G. S., J. E. Smialek, and W. G. Troutman. Sudden Death in Adolescents from the Inhalation of Typewriter Correction Fluid. *Journal of the American Medical Association*, **253**:1604–1606, 1985.

Schwartz, R. H. Deliberate Inhalation of Isobutyl Nitrite during Adolescence: A Descriptive Study. *National Institute of Drug Abuse Monograph Series*, **83**:81–85, 1988.

Chapter 29

Milhorn, H. T., Jr. Anabolic Steroids: Another Form of Drug Abuse. *Journal of the Mississippi State Medical Association*, **32**:293–297, 1991.

Milhorn, H. T., Jr. *Chemical Dependence: Diagnosis, Treatment, and Prevention.* Springer-Verlag, New York, 1990.

Tsuang, J. W. Psychiatric Complications and Dependence Potential of Anabolic Steroids. *Family Practice Recertification*, **15**:67–73, 1993.

Chapter 30

Barnes, D. M. New Data Intensify the Agony over Ecstasy. *Science*, **239**:864–866, 1988.

Brown, R. T. and N. J. Braden. Hallucinogens. *Pediatric Clinics of North America*, **34**:341–347, 1987.

Schwartz, R. H. and D. E. Smith. Hallucinogenic Mushrooms. *Clinical Pediatrics*, **27**:70–73, 1988.

Strassman, R. J. Adverse Reaction to Psychedelic Drugs: A Review of the Literature. *Journal of Nervous and Mental Disease*, **172**:572–578, 1984.

Index